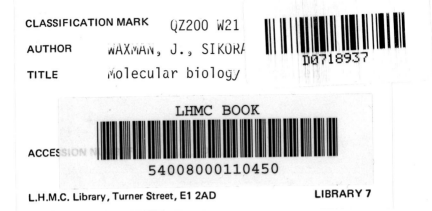

THE MOLECULAR BIOLOGY
OF CANCER

THE MOLECULAR BIOLOGY OF CANCER

EDITED BY

JONATHAN WAXMAN
MD BSc MRCP
Senior Lecturer in Clinical Oncology
Royal Postgraduate Medical School
Hammersmith Hospital
London

KAROL SIKORA
PhD FRCP FRCR
Professor of Clinical Oncology
Royal Postgraduate Medical School
Hammersmith Hospital
London

BLACKWELL SCIENTIFIC PUBLICATIONS

OXFORD LONDON EDINBURGH

BOSTON MELBOURNE

© 1989 by
Blackwell Scientific Publications
Editorial offices:
Osney Mead, Oxford OX2 0EL
 (*Orders*: Tel. 0865–240201)
8 John Street, London WC1N 2ES
23 Ainslie Place, Edinburgh EH3 6AJ
3 Cambridge Center, Suite 208
 Cambridge, Massachusetts 02142, USA
107 Barry Street, Carlton
 Victoria 3053, Australia

First published 1989

Set by Enset (Photosetting) Ltd
Midsomer Norton, Bath, Avon
Printed and bound in Great Britain
at The University Press, Cambridge

DISTRIBUTORS

USA
 Year Book Medical Publishers
 200 North LaSalle Street,
 Chicago, Illinois 60601
 (*Orders*: Tel. 312–726–9733)

Canada
 The C.V. Mosby Company
 5240 Finch Avenue East
 Scarborough, Ontario
 (*Orders*: Tel. 416–298–1588)

Australia
 Blackwell Scientific Publications
 (Australia) Pty Ltd
 107 Barry Street
 Carlton, Victoria 3053
 (*Orders*: Tel. 03–347–0300)

British Library
Cataloguing in Publication Data

Molecular biology of cancer.
 1. Man. Cancer. Molecular biology
 I. Waxman, Jonathan   II. Sikora,
 Karol
 616.99'407

ISBN 0–632–01977–8

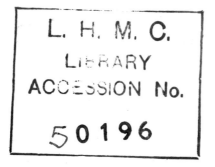

CONTENTS

LIST OF CONTRIBUTORS

D.N. CARNEY MB, MH, PhD, FRCP
Consultant Physician, Mater Misericordiae Hospital, Dublin.

A.G. DALGLEISH MB, FRACP, MRCP
Senior Lecturer and Honorary Consultant, Clinical Research Centre, Northwick Park Hospital, Harrow.

A.A. EPENETOS PhD, MRCP
Consultant and Senior Lecturer in Clinical Oncology, Imperial Cancer Research Fund Oncology Group, Royal Postgraduate Medical School, Hammersmith Hospital, London.

P.J. FARRELL MA, PhD
Director, Ludwig Institute, St Mary's Hospital Medical School, London.

W.J. GULLICK PhD
Head, Imperial Cancer Research Fund Molecular Oncology Laboratories, Hammersmith Hospital, London.

H. KALOFONOS MD
Research Fellow in Clinical Oncology, Imperial Cancer Research Fund Oncology Group, Royal Postgraduate Medical School, Hammersmith Hospital, London.

K. SIKORA PhD, FRCR, FRCP
Professor of Clinical Oncology, Department of Clinical Oncology, Royal Postgraduate Medical School, Hammersmith Hospital, London.

G.B. SIVOLAPENKO BSc
Research Fellow in Clinical Oncology and Immunology, Imperial Cancer Research Fund Oncology Group and Department of Immunology, Royal Postgraduate Medical School, Hammersmith Hospital, London.

H. THOMAS MA, MRCP
Registrar, Department of Clinical Oncology, Royal Postgraduate Medical School, Hammersmith Hospital, London.

J. TIDY BSc, MBBS
Research Fellow, Ludwig Institute, St Mary's Hospital Medical School, London.

J. V. WATSON MSc, MD, DMRT, FRCR
Consultant, Medical Research Council Oncology Unit, The Medical School, Cambridge.

J. WAXMAN MD, BSc, MRCP
Senior Lecturer and Honorary Consultant, Department of Clinical Oncology, Royal Postgraduate Medical School, Hammersmith Hospital, London.

J. O. WHITE PhD
Senior Lecturer in Obstetrics and Gynaecology, Institute of Obstetrics and Gynaecology, Royal Postgraduate Medical School, Hammersmith Hospital, London.

D. J. VENTER MB, ChB
Research Fellow, Ludwig Institute, Middlesex Hospital, London.

PREFACE

WITHIN THE last decade, there have been remarkable developments in our understanding of the molecular processes of malignancy. This is a time of excitement for oncology, a time when we are
able to recognise the specific molecular changes within the genome
that cause cellular transformation. We are at the brink of applying this
new understanding to the treatment of people with cancer, so that it
may soon be possible to tailor treatments specifically, selectively
inhibiting the growth of each patient's tumour. These developments
have proceeded at such a speed that the clinician is left slightly dazed,
peering through the smoke of science's slipstream. There is a need for
these scientific advances to be translated into an intelligible form for
the clinician who is to apply them, and this is the aim of *The Molecular
Biology Of Cancer*.

Jonathan Waxman
Karol Sikora

1 ONCOGENES AND CANCER

H. THOMAS AND J. WAXMAN

THE DEVELOPMENT of molecular biology has led to an understanding of the molecular processes of cancer. These advances have brought us to the threshold of describing details of the evolution of tumours and their controlling mechanisms. This chapter provides an overview of the techniques of molecular biology which have resulted in these discoveries and describes the role of oncogenes and growth factors in malignancy.

THE TECHNIQUES OF MOLECULAR BIOLOGY

We are now able to comprehend details of changes in the molecular structure of the nucleic acids. The techniques by which these changes are analysed are briefly summarised below.

Preparation of DNA

Nucleic acids are stable structures which can be extracted from fresh material or tissue that has been 'fixed' and stored. The first steps in this process involve cell homogenisation, and the separation of DNA from cellular debris first by extraction in phenol and then by precipitation in ethanol. In order to analyse the sequences of bases within specific segments of DNA, the crude preparation is subjected to further fragmentation by the use of restriction endonucleases. Restriction endonucleases are naturally occurring enzymes first isolated from bacteria. There are at least 300 restriction endonucleases and they function in host protection against virus invasion and in nucleic acid repair by cleaving DNA at the site of specific base sequences. The use of these enzymes allows the preparation of DNA fragments with common terminal sequences. The cleaved DNA has exposed 'sticky ends', created by the endonuclease, and these single strands can be hybridised with compatible DNA fragments (Table 1.1).

Table 1.1 Commonly used restriction endonucleases and their sequence specificities

Enzyme	Sequence cleaved
I *Bam*Hl	G GATCC CCTAG G
II *Bg*II	GCCNNNN NGGC CGGN NNNNCCG
I *Eco*RI	G AATTC CTTAA G
III *Hind*III	A AGCTT TTCGA A
I *Pst*I	CTGCA G G ACGTC
I *Taq*I	T CGA AGC T

Gene cloning

Further analysis may be performed after the production of multiple copies of prepared DNA fragments by gene cloning. Multiple replicas are synthesised by insertion of DNA fragments into a bacterial genome using a plasmid, bacteriophage or cosmid vector. The simplest technique involves the use of plasmids, which are cellular parasites, that confer antibiotic resistance to host bacteria. The prepared fragments of DNA to be analysed are integrated into plasmid DNA by the use of restriction enzymes that cleave circular DNA. By altering the local environment, the circle of plasmid DNA is closed, incorporating a fragment of the 'foreign' DNA into the plasmid genome. Following this, sucrose gradient centrifugation is performed and used to select plasmids of specific molecular weight for further investigation. Next, plasmids containing these specific DNA inserts are introduced into host *Escherichia coli*, where they replicate. Included within the plasmid is an antibiotic resistance gene, so that only *E. coli* bearing plasmids containing the DNA fragments under investigation will grow on nutrient media containing antibiotic. By this means, multiple copies of single DNA fragments from a preparation of interest can be obtained in significant amounts.

Genomic libraries

This collection of DNA fragments is termed a genomic library. However, in the natural state many of the random fragments prepared will not be actively transcribed into messenger RNA (mRNA). More relevant to a biological analysis is the preparation of a complimentary DNA (cDNA) library, in which only those 'functional' sequences transcribed into mRNA are copied. This technique involves the initial extraction of mRNA rather than DNA. Functional mRNA has a polyadenylated 3' terminal and can be extracted on an oligo-deoxythymidine affinity column. Using reverse transcriptase, extracted mRNA can then be used to produce double stranded DNA, which can be inserted into the appropriate vector and cloned. By this means, a cDNA library is prepared containing functional DNA alone.

Structural analysis

Further examination of the structure of DNA is performed by the technique ot Southern blotting. DNA fragments are separated by electrophoresis on an agarose gel. After electrophoresis, the DNA is exposed to alkali to produce single stranded fragments. The denatured DNA is then 'blotted' onto a sheet of nitrocellulose which is laid over the gel. These blotted single strands of DNA are exposed to prepared single stranded copies of the cDNA from a genomic library into which p32 has been incorporated. Hybridisation occurs between complimentary strands of DNA. The 'blotted' sheet is washed and dried, and placed against a photographic film. The radioactive DNA corresponding to the gene of interest will then be seen as a defined band on the film. In Northern blotting, p32 DNA fragments are hybridised to RNA. (Fig. 1.1.). In Western blotting 'staining' is by means of an antibody directed against a protein product of a specific gene.

VIRUSES AND CANCER

The significance of viruses in the aetiology of animal cancers has been known since the beginning of the century when Peyton Rous estab-

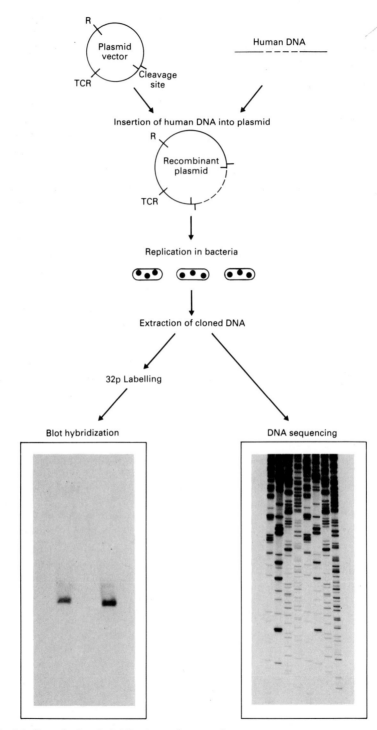

Fig. 1.1. Gene cloning, hybridisation and sequencing.

lished that a filterable infective agent caused sarcomas in chickens, and Ellerman and Bang described erythroblastosis in chickens. Further evidence for a viral cause for cancers came in the 1940s when Bittner described a 'B particle' transmitted in maternal milk, which caused a 'hereditable' breast cancer in rodents. More recently, viruses have been linked to the development of human tumours: Epstein–Barr virus has been associated with Burkitt's lymphoma and naso-pharyngeal cancer; hepatitis B virus with hepatoma; papilloma viruses with genital tract malignancy; and the immunodeficiency virus with AIDS related tumours. Oncogenic viruses are classified according to whether they contain DNA or RNA in their genome. DNA tumour viruses include hepatitis B, papilloma and Epstein–Barr and are thought to be the major cause of human viral induced cancers. RNA tumour viruses are at present not thought to be a major cause of human cancers, and the only known associations are between HIV1 and 2 and AIDS related malignancies, and HTLV1 and T cell lymphoma/leukaemia. However, it is the RNA viruses which cause malignancy in animals that have been subject to the greatest study because their genome is less complex and relatively easier to investigate than that of the DNA viruses (Table 1.2). Within each RNA virus genome, there are three gene sequences,

Table 1.2 Examples of viral oncogenes, their cellular counterparts and associated human malignancies

Oncogene	Animal tumour	Human gene	Human tumour
v-*src*	Chicken sarcoma	s-*src*	
v-*ras*	Rat sarcoma	c-*ras* (Ha & Ki)	Bladder carcinoma Colorectal adenoca Ovarian adenoca
v-*myc*	Chicken leukaemia	c-*myc*	Prostate carcinoma Breast carcinoma
		(L-*myc*)	Lung carcinoma
		(N-*myc*)	Neuroblastoma
v-*erb*B	Chicken erythroblastosis	c-*erb*B1	Brain tumour
		c-*erb*B2	Breast cancer
v-*erb*A	Avian erythroblastosis	c-*erb*A	Breast carcinoma
v-*sis*	Monkey sarcoma	c-*sis*	Brain tumour (high-grade)
v-*abl*	Mouse leukaemia	c-*abl*	Chronic myeloid leukaemia

'*gag*', '*pol*' and '*env*'. The *pol* gene encodes reverse transcriptase enzymes which convert viral RNA into DNA. This is then incorporated into the host genome. *Gag* and *env* encode proteins that package the viral RNA produced by the host after viral transfection.

Analysis of the genome of oncogenic viruses has revealed that viruses capable of transformation have lost their replicative genes. In their place are nucleic acid sequences termed v-*onc* which confer malignant potential. These substituted sequences are termed oncogenes. Each retroviral oncogene has a three letter notation specific to the virus from which it was first isolated. Remarkably, oncogenic sequences present in viruses are found to be conserved throughout eukaryotic evolution and present in many normal hosts that are tumour free. The normal cellular counterparts of viral oncogenes are termed c-*onc*. The presence of oncogenes in the normal genome suggests either a possible non-malignant function of these genes or their incorporation during evolution as a result of viral infection.

There are many different theories as to the molecular origins of malignancy. Tumour development is thought to follow oncogene activation. Oncogene activation may follow from the gene re-arrangement that occurs for c-*abl* in leukaemia or point mutation, as described for the *ras* oncogene in human bladder cancer. Virus infection or mutation may lead to the insertion of a viral promoter or enhancer into the cell genome, activating an existing oncogene. Oncogenes may produce an abnormal protein product that causes abnormal regulation of cell growth.

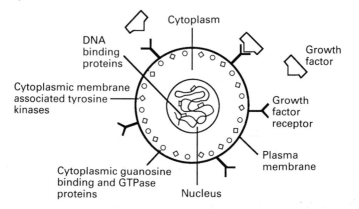

Fig. 1.2   Sites of action of oncogene products in different areas of the mammalian cell.

Within the cell there are a number of levels at which the protein products of oncogenes might have effect (Fig. 1.2). In the nucleus, oncogene products such as those of c-*myc* and c-*myb* can lead to increased gene expression. Oncogene proteins function in the cell cytoplasm either by having tyrosine kinase activity as do *src* oncogenes or by their GTPase activity such as the *ras* oncogenes (Fig. 1.3). Finally, some oncogene products could act at the level of the cell surface as is the case with the epidermal growth factor receptor. Several other peptide growth factor receptors are likely to be oncogene products. The level of receptor expression determines the behaviour of a cell in the presence of the relevant growth factors. Abnormal expression of receptor or increased affinity can lead to malignancy.

ONCOGENES AND THEIR PRODUCTS IN SPECIFIC MALIGNANT DISEASES

Descriptions of the involvement of oncogenes in human cancer are a recent phenomenon. The techniques of molecular biology have been applied to a wide variety of human tumours and in a proportion of patients with specific malignant diseases specific molecular changes have been noted. The significance of these changes is firstly in ascribing the

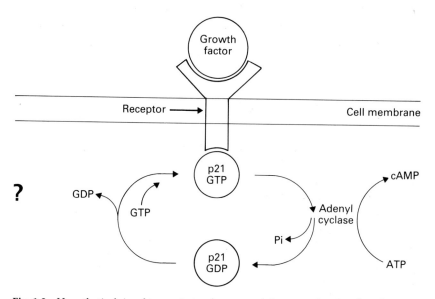

Fig. 1.3 Hypothetical signal transmission from growth factor to adenyl cyclase through p21 and growth factor receptor.

origins of malignancy to a viral cause and secondly in the possibility of designing treatments for malignancy, tailored to the molecular basis of each individual's disease. In this next section, we review for the clinician the role of oncogenes in the main human tumours.

COLORECTAL CANCER

The techniques of molecular biology have been applied to colorectal cancer in order to establish the incidence and clinical correlates of oncogene expression. Work in this field is at an early stage. However, a number of observations have been defined and controversies established.

Work on individuals, and subsequently families, with familial adenomatous polyposis has located the gene for this condition to chromosome 5 [1]. In individuals with sporadic colorectal carcinomas at least 20% are found to lose one of the alleles on chromosome 5 which is present in normal matched tissue [2]. These findings support Knudson's contention that the mutation for a dominantly inherited cancer susceptibility may be the first stage in a recessive change in the tumour cells, with sporadic and inherited forms arising in the same gene; that mutations act recessively at the cellular level; and that both copies of the gene must be lost for the cancer to develop [3, 4].

Proto-oncogene abnormalitities have been described in colorectal cancer. The most commonly reported observation concerns the c-*myc* oncogene. C-*myc* is the oncogene of the avian leukosis virus, which in chickens lead to the development of myelocytomas, lymphomas, sarcomas and carcinomas. The protein product of the c-*myc* oncogene is a molecular weight 62 000 peptide, which functions as a transmembrane-acting regulator of transcription.

The aberrant expression of the c-*myc* proto-oncogene observed in colorectal cancer may result from molecular changes at different levels. It is not clear whether the abnormal levels of c-*myc* mRNA and the c-*myc* protein seen in this malignancy are related to gene amplification or increased transcription. The exact incidence of c-*myc* proto-oncogene abnormalities is variably reported. In one series of 45 patients, three had c-*myc* amplification [5]. In a group of 15 patients, 12 had increased c-*myc* expression without evidence of gene amplification [6]. In a further series of 29 patients, 21 had increased expression of c-*myc* and none of the tumours had c-*myc* amplification [7]. When tumour and normal mucosa from the same patient were contrasted, expression of c-*myc* was found to be increased up to 40-fold in malignant as compared to normal surrounding colonic mucosa. It is of interest that levels of mRNA expression of c-*myc* mRNA and of p62 c-*myc* protein are found to be directly correlated with the degree of differentiation of the tumour. Well differentiated colorectal cancers had the highest levels of mRNA expression and of protein production [8]. Using an antibody to synthetic peptide fragments of the p62 product, variable immunostaining is seen in cancer as compared to rectal polyps and normal colonic mucosa. In normal mucosa the staining is greatest in the mid-zone of the crypts. In polyps, the most intense staining is seen in dysplastic areas. C-*myc* expression has been examined in primary tumours and compared with secondary deposits in the same patient. A two- to tenfold increase in transcription was found and the levels of increase found to be the same in both primary and secondary tumours in the same patient [8] (Fig. 1.4).

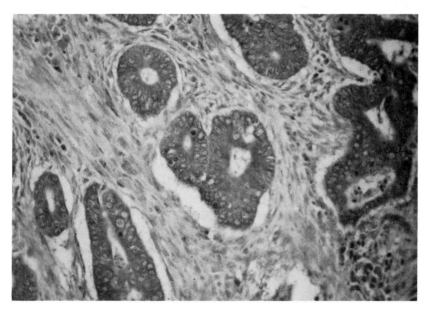

Fig. 1.4. C-*myc* expression in a primary colonic tumour demonstrated by staining with a monoclonal antibody to c-*myc* protein.

Other proto-oncogenes have been assessed in colorectal cancer. It has been found that both c-*fos* and N-*myc* are not expressed [9]. Ha-*ras* expression has been examined in mucin and non-mucin secreting cell lines and Ha-*ras* expression found to be five-fold increased in mucin secreting, but not expressed in non-mucin secreting cell lines [10]. Ki-*ras* and Ha-*ras* oncogene expression was assessed in 12 patients with colorectal cancer and found to be increased up to 20-fold. Unlike the situation with c-*myc* expression, there was no correlation with tumour stage or differentiation [11].

LUNG CANCER

Oncogene abnormalities have been assessed in lung cancer, and attempts made to establish clinical correlates. The most consistently observed abnormalities relate to the *myc* family of oncogenes. Most investigations have been performed on small cell lung cancer and this relates to the ease with which this tumour is successfully grown in cell culture.

Unlike colorectal cancer where abnormalities of gene expression are reported, in lung cancer gene amplification is a more common feature. The most common cytogenic abnormality described is a structural change in chromosome 3, where the lesion is a deletion of the short arm [12]. However, L-*myc* has been mapped to chromosome 1 [13]. Forty-four small cell lung cancer cell lines were established from 227 patients and differences in L-*myc* amplification assessed in patients on presentation and at relapse of their illness. Two of 19 lines established from primary tumours had DNA amplification as compared with 11 of 25 established from relapsed tumours [14]. In another study 19 of 45 patients had increased amplification of either n-*myc* or c-*myc* in the primary tumour. Examination of metastatic tumour showed an increase in copy number as compared to the primary tumour in the same patient, which the authors suggest is an initiating event allowing for the development of metastases [15]. Amplification of the proto-oncogene L-*myc* may be increased up to 20-fold increased in small cell lung cancer cell lines [16].

Although the p62 c-*myc* product is normally nuclear, radio-labelled antibodies raised to p62 c-*myc* peptide fragments may be used for tumour localisation. Why scanning using these antibodies should be successful is not clear, but may relate to tumour necrosis with local release of p62 c-*myc* protein from its nuclear site. Iodine-131 labelled antibody was used in an attempt to localise tumour in 20 patients with different malignant diseases. Only in patients with lung cancer, was the imaging successful and in 12 of 14 patients with carcinoma of the bronchus uptake of labelled antibody correlated with pulmonary change evident on plain X-ray [16].

A number of growth factors have been shown to stimulate the growth of lung cancer cells in culture, and these include insulin-like growth factor 1 (somatomedin C) and bombesin. These growth factors have normal and abnormal regulatory function. IGF1 is a peptide hormone, that mediates growth hormone activity. IGF1 levels were measured in normal and neoplastic tissue from ten specimens of resected lung in patients with non-small cell lung cancer. IGF1 concentrations were signficantly higher in neoplastic as compared to normal tissue [17]. Bombesin is a 14 amino acid peptide first isolated from frog skin. Intravenous injection of bombesin stimulates the secretion of gut hormones, prolactin, growth hormone and insulin. The human counterpart of bombesin, gastrin releasing peptide, has recently been isolated and is a 27 amino acid peptide. Receptors for bombesin/gastrin releasing peptide have been found in normal infant lung and in small cell lung cancer. Bombesin/gastrin releasing peptide stimulates the growth of small cell lung cancer cells in culture, by up to 150-fold. Bombesin/gastrin releasing peptide has no stimulatory effect on non-small cell lung cancer lines. Antibodies to bombesin inhibit the growth of small cell lung cancer xenografts in nude mice. This is discussed in more detail in Chapter 4.

NEUROBLASTOMA

Gross chromosomal changes in neuroblastoma are well known. The most consistent observations are of the presence of 'double minutes' and 'homogeneously staining regions'. In 70% of patients abnormalities are seen in the short arm of chromosome 1. In 1983, Schwab noted amplification of a c-*myc* related sequence which he described as N-*myc* and this change occurred in 30% of patients with neuroblastoma where amplification may be increased three- to 300-fold. [18]. N-*myc* has been mapped to the homogeneously staining regions of a number of different chromosomes in neuroblastoma cell lines and is mapped to chromosome 2p band 23–24 in normal cells [19]. N-*myc* amplification is also found in retinoblastoma and small cell lung cancer. The N-*myc* gene has been sequenced and consists of three exons, the first of which consists of 637 nucleotides: the second and third exons encode for peptide products containing 255 and 201 amino acids respectively. There is partial sequence homology between the c-*myc* and n-*myc* oncogene with 30% of the coding domains of these two oncogenes having a close structural relationship [20].

In patients with neuroblastoma hyperdiploidy is common in early stage tumours but not in the more advanced malignancies. N-*myc* amplification is found in late stage tumours which tend to be pseudodiploid or hypotriploid [21]. N-*myc* amplification is elevated at the same level, within different parts of the same tumour as shown by an analysis of 30 different nueroblastomas. In patients who have relapsed the N-*myc* copy number is consistently the same as shown in serial samples of tumour taken from 25 patients [19]. It may be that antibodies raised to the protein product of N-*myc* could be used in tumour imaging and ultimately in treatment. Antibodies have been raised against the protein product of the clone pNb-1 derived from a neuroblastoma cell line [22], but have not yet entered clinical use.

PROSTATE CANCER

The importance of cellular oncogenes in the development of prostate cancer has been the subject of only limited investigation, despite the importance of this disease as the second most common malignancy of man in the Western world. The level of c-*myc* transcription in prostate cancer and hypertrophy has been compared. C-*myc* expression was assessed by densitometric scanning of Northern gels. C-*myc* RNA levels were twice as high in seven patients with prostatic cancer as eight patients with benign hypertrophy. There was considerable overlap between the groups, the study was small and there seemed to be no direct correlation between c-*myc* expression and stage and grade of malignancy [23].

An immunochemical assay was used to measure the expression of the *ras* oncogene protein p21 in 19 patients with benign hypertrophy and 29 patients with prostatic cancer and compared with 'normal' prostatic tissue. Normal and hypertrophic prostate tissue did not stain with the p21 antibody. Prostatic tissue from 23 of 29 patients with prostatic cancer stained for p21. Staining was related to histological grade and was positive in all 17 undifferentiated tumours, but in only six of 12 patients with more differentiated tumours [24].

A number of different probes were used to assess oncogene expression in human prostatic carcinoma cell lines. Each of the cell lines examined expressed a number of different oncogenes and the level of transcription varied between these lines. The oncogenes expressed most commonly included Ha-*ras*, Ki-*ras*, n-*ras*, c-*myc*, c-*fos*, c-*myb*, c-*fms* and c-*sis*. One interesting finding concerned the androgen sensitive PC82 cell line. Androgen withdrawal was accompanied by ten-fold reduction in *fos* mRNA and a two-fold reduction in Ha-*ras* mRNA transcription. These changes were maximal two weeks after withdrawal of androgen and were unaccompanied by the change in c-*myc* expression. These findings are difficult to assess and may simply represent a non-specific change accompanying the reduction in cell growth that follows androgen withdrawal. Alternatively, it may be that androgens induce cellular oncogene expression which is the primary event leading to abnormal proliferation [25].

Steroid hormones, prolactin and growth hormone are involved in the stimulation of growth of the normal human prostate. A specific, prostate growth promoting peptide has been isolated from normal rat prostatic tissue. This peptide has a molecular weight of 25 000 and has mitogenic activity. The significance of this finding in relation to human prostate cancer is unknown.

BRAIN TUMOURS

C-*erb*B1 is the human homologue of the transforming oncogene of the avian erythroblastosis virus which causes erythroid leukaemia and sarcomas in chickens, and in man has been mapped to chromosome 7. C-*erb*B1 encodes for three of the four domains of the epidermal growth factor receptor. This receptor in normal humans consists of an external binding domain, a transmembrane domain and two cytoplasmic domains that have tyrosine kinase activity. Epidermal growth factor receptor activation leads to a voltage independent calcium flux, and alterations in amino acid, nucleotide and glucose transport with changes in protein phosphorylation and ultimately decreased synthesis of DNA. Epidermal growth factor is found in the natural state in human milk and is excreted into the urinary tract. Epidermal growth factor was first isolated in 1962 from the mouse submandibular gland.

C-*sis* is the transforming oncogene of the simian sarcoma virus which causes sarcomas in monkeys. C-*sis* has been mapped to chromosome 22 and encodes for a peptide of molecular weight 28 000 called p28. P28 has structural homology with platelet derived growth factor. Most low grade brain tumours such as neuromas, angiomas and meningiomas were thought to have a normal karyotype. However, detailed analysis shows monosomy or gene loss of chromosomes 22 [25] with trisomy of chromosome 7 in up to 75% of tumours [26]. High grade tumours such as malignant gliomas, in contrast have an abnormal chromosomal complement and over 50% have over-representation of chromosome 7 [25, 26]. It is tempting, therefore, to associate malignant brain tumours with c-*erb* and c-*sis* oncogene activation. In this context, it is of interest that gliomas grown in culture have frequently been reported to secrete PDGF, and that human gliomas express epidermal growth factor receptor.

N-*myc* amplification and overexpression has been reported in neuroblastoma, retinoblastoma, and small cell lung carcinoma, which are all tumours of neural crest origin. N-*myc* amplification is also reported in astrocytoma [27].

The possible application of these observations is to tumour localisation and treatment. Radio-labelled antibody to the EGF receptor has been injected into the carotid artery and uptake of antibody correlated with the anatomical site of tumour. Iodine-131 labelled antibody has been used in a few patients to treat EGF expressing brain tumours. This method may allow higher 'sterilising' dosages of radiotherapy to be delivered to the tumour with reduced likelihood of damage to normal tissues.

Growth factor production has been observed in the human brain tumours. Several glioma lines have been found to secrete platelet derived growth factor or a platelet derived growth factor-like molecule. As a result, several groups of workers are investigating the possibility of inhibiting the growth of gliomas by use of antibodies to PDGF. This work is at a preliminary stage.

BLADDER CANCER

Bladder cancer was among the first of the major malignancies in which oncogene activation was shown to be significant. In early work, oncogenic potential was assessed by the ability of DNA fragments prepared from tumours to transform NIH/3T3 fibroblasts. Using this approach, oncogenes of the *ras* gene family have been found to be the most commonly detected abnormally activated oncogene group. There are at least five members of the *ras* family which take their name from v-Ha-*ras* , the transforming oncogene of the Harvey murine sarcoma virus. This oncogene encodes for a protein of molecular weight 21 000, p21, which has sequence homology with guanidine nucleotide binding proteins. These proteins are involved in metabolic pathways where signals, elicited by ligand binding to membrane receptor, are translated into changes in intracellular metabolism mediated by protein kinases. H-*ras* activation has been found to be due most commonly to point mutations in codons 12 or 61. However, other point mutations have been detected in codons 13, 59 and 63. These base changes lead to structural alterations in the *ras* protein product.

Transfection studies have shown that the DNA from a proportion of patients with bladder cancer has transforming activity which is due to activation of Ha-*ras*. The proportion of patients having *ras* activation is small: approximately 10% [28, 29]. A significant proportion of patients with bladder cancer have chromosomal changes and five of 12 (42%) previously untreated patients had a deletion of the short arm of chromosome 11 [30]. Work with bladder cancer grown in culture shows similar gross chromosomal change which was first demonstrated for the human EJ tumour line [31]. In humans, Ha-*ras* is localised to the distal end of the short arm of chromosome 11 [32], suggesting that homozygosity of translocation allows for the abnormal expression of activated oncogene.

There is a clear association between exposure to chemical carcinogens and the later development of bladder cancer, as shown for workers in the dye and rubber industries. It may be that this exposure leads to oncogene activation, as has been demonstrated for Ha-*ras* with anti-BPDB the carcinogenic metabolite of benzopyrene [33].

Activated Ha-*ras* has only been found in a proportion of patients with bladder cancer and the significance of this finding in relation to the majority of patients is unknown. More detailed studies are required, correlating oncogene expression with carcinogen exposure and tumour stage and grade.

Large quantities of epidermal growth factor are found in human urine and are thought to be secreted by renal tubular cells. The physiological role of epidermal growth factor is unknown. The effects of epidermal growth factor on normal urothelium and transitional cell carcinoma has been tested. Growth stimulation and ornithine decarboxylase activity in response to epidermal growth factor has been examined in cell lines. All four transitional cell carcinoma cell lines but only one of four urothelial lines were stimulated in a dose related fashion by epidermal growth factor. The significance of this finding is not known [34].

BREAST CANCER

Application of the techniques of molecular biology has led to the identification of specific molecular changes in breast cancer. The most important observations concern the epidermal growth factor receptor and the steroid hormone receptor. Recently the gene coding for the oestrogen receptor has been cloned and sequenced. There is extensive homology between oestrogen receptor cDNA and the v-erbA gene of the avian erythroblastosis virus [35]. The progesterone receptor has been cloned too and mapped to chromosome band 11q13 [36]. Using a monoclonal antibody raised against the EGF receptor, 104 primary breast tumours and 14 lymph node secondaries were examined. Thirty-five of the 104 tumours had detectable EGF receptor. Fifty-three of these tumours contained oestrogen receptor (51%), but only four (8%) of these oestrogen receptor positive tumours contain EGF receptor. In contrast, 31 of 51 (61%) ER negative tumours contained receptor and so there seemed to be an inverse relationship between EGF and oestrogen receptor positivity. Ten of 14 of the lymph node metastases (71%) contain EGF receptors. The authors suggested that the presence of EGF receptor is associated with metastatic potential and correlated with a reduced likelihood of hormone sensitivity [37]. One of the most interesting observations in experimental models of breast cancer has been the finding in the MCF-7 cell line, which is a human, post-menopausal, hormone sensitive, breast cancer line, that transfection of the oncogene v-ras confers oestradiol independence [38].

Abnormalities in c-myc and Ha-ras expression have been examined in breast cancer. In 100 patients with breast cancer, no point mutations were observed in the H-ras oncogene [39]. Levels of the p21 H-ras protein product have been assessed by a quantitative method which compared tissue from 15 patients with tumours from five patients with fibrocystic disease. In the patients with fibrocystic disease absolute levels of p21 were less than 5 pg/mg of protein. Ten of the patients with cancer had greater than 10 pg of p21/ug of protein [40]. C-myc expression was examined in 120 primary breast cancers; in 39 patients, c-myc was amplified, and amplification tended to correlate with increased patient age [41].

Breast cancer cell lines are dependent upon steroidal and peptide growth factors. The effects of oestrogenic steroids, androgens, and glucocorticoids are established. However, the significance of peptide growth factors such as epidermal growth factor, IGF1 and 2, and transforming growth factors A and B have only recently become known. IGF1 may be a significant autocrine growth factor in human hormone independent breast cancer cell lines. A comparison of two oestrogen independent lines with two oestrogen unresponsive lines showed two- to ten-fold higher levels of IGF1 production in the independent lines [42]. Breast cancer cell lines secrete platelet derived growth factor (PDGF) [43]. PDGF is a powerful mitogen, which may enable cells to respond to other growth factors. It may be that the production of PDGF by breast cancer is significant in mediating the effects of paracrine agents. In the MDA 468 human breast cancer cell line the EGF receptor is overexpressed as a result of gene amplification. Each tumour cell has approximately two million receptors and the cell line responds to EGF by growth inhibition. The mechanism for growth inhibition has been investigated using a monoclonal antibody to EGF receptor. It has been shown that down-regulation of the receptor by EGF results from an increased rate of receptor degradation rather than decreased receptor synthesis [44]. Transforming growth factor beta is a fibroblast growth factor. Exposure of the MDA 468 cell line to TGF-B in the presence of epidermal growth factor enhances EGF-receptor mRNA accumulation. Altered EGF receptor expression affects the cells response to EGF and ultimately leads to inhibition of growth. The results of this work suggest that the inhibitory effects of TGF-B in this cell line are mediated by means of modulation of EGF receptor gene expression [45].

CONCLUSIONS

The development of the techniques of molecular biology and its application to human tumours is still at an early stage. A considerable amount of work needs to be done in correlating the presence of oncogenes and mutated oncogenes, their products and absolute levels of their product's expression with tumour stage and prognosis. The prospect for the oncologist is a remarkable advance in tumour staging using antibodies to peptide products of oncogenes. Arguably the best future scenario for the treatment of malignancy involves the possibility of tumour transfection with genes capable of switching off malignant growth, and that these transfected genes would themselves be switched on by normal regulatory hormones present in the patient's circulation. By this means, viral infection could be used to control the process of viral oncogenesis.

REFERENCES

1 Bodmer, W.F., Bailey, C.J., Bodmer, J. *et al.* Localisation of the gene for familial adenomatous polyposis on chromosome 5. *Nature.* 1987, **328**: 614–616.

2 Solomon, E., Voss, R., Hall, V. *et al*. Chromosome 5 allele loss in human colorectal carcinomas. *Nature*. 1987, **328**: 616–619.

3 Knudson. A.G. Genetics of Human Cancer. *Annu Rev Genet*. 1986, **20**: 231–251.

4 Knudson, A.G. Mutation and cancer: statistical study of retinoblastoma. *Proc Natl Acad Sci USA*. 1971, **68(4)**: 820–3.

5 Meltzer, S.J., Ahenen, D.J., Battifora, H., Yokoto, J. and Cline, M.J. Protooncogene abnormalities in colon cancers and adenomatous polyps. *Gastroenterology*. 1987, **92**: 1174–1180.

6 Sikora, K., Chan, S., Evan, G. *et al*. C-myc oncogene expression in colorectal cancer. *Cancer*. 1986, **59**: 1289–1295.

7 Erisman, M.D., Rothberg, P.G., Diehl, R.E. *et al*. Deregulation of c-myc gene expression in human colon carcinoma is not accompanied by amplification or rearrangement of the gene. *Mol Cell Biol*. 1985, **5**: 1969–1976.

8 Tsuboi, K., Hirayoshi, K., Takeuchi, K. *et al*. Expression of the c-myc gene in human gastrointestinal malignancies. *Biochem Biophys Res Commun*. 1987, **146**: 699–704.

9 Alexander, R.J., Buxbaum, J.N and Raicht, R.F. Oncogene alterations in primary human colon tumours. *Gastroenterology*. 1986, **91**: 1503–1510.

10 Augenlicht, L.H., Augeron, C., Yander, G. and Laboisse, C. Overexpression of ras in mucus-secreting human colon carcinoma cells of low tumorigenicity. *Cancer Res*. 1987, **47**: 3763–3765.

11 Kerr, I.B., Spandidos, D.A., Finlay, I.G. *et al*. The relation of ras family oncogene expression to conventional staging criteria and clinical outcome in colorectal carcinoma. *Br J Cancer*. 1986, **53**: 231–235.

12 Morstyn, G., Brown, J., Novak, U. *et al*. Heterogeneous cytogentic abnormalities in small cell lung cancer cell lines. *Cancer Res*. 1987, **47**: 3322–3327.

13 Nau, M.M., Brookes, B.J., Battey, J. *et al*. L-myc, a new myc-related gene amplified and expressed in human small cell lung cancer. *Nature*. 1985, **318**: 69–73.

14 Johnson, B.E., Ihde, D.C., Makuch, R.W. *et al*. Myc family oncogene amplification in tumour cell lines established from small cell lung cancer patients and its relationship to clinical status and course. *J Clin Invest*. 1987, **79**: 1629–1634.

15 Wong, A.J., Ruppert, J.M., Eggleston, J. *et al*. Gene amplification of lung cancer by a radiolabelled monoclonal antibody against the c-myc oncogene product. *Science*. 1986, **25**: 461–464.

16 Chan, S.Y.T., Evan, G.I., Ritson, A. *et al*. Localisation of lung cancer by a radiolabelled monoclonal antibody against the c-myc oncogene product. *Br J Cancer*. 1986, **54**: 761–769.

17 Siefter, E.J., Sausville, E.A. and Battey, J. Comparison of amplified and unamplified c-myc gene structure and expression in human small cell lung carcinoma cell lines. *Cancer Res*. 1986, **46**: 2050–2055.

18 Schwab, M., Alitalo, K., Klempnaeur, K.H., *et al*. Amplified DNA with limited homology to myc cellular oncogene is shared by human neuroblastoma cell lines and a neuroblastoma tumour. *Nature*. 1983, **305**: 245–248.

19 Brodeur, G.M., Hayes, F.A., Green, A.A. *et al*. Consistent N-myc copy number in simultaneous or consecutive neuroblastoma samples from sixty individual patients. *Cancer Res*. 1987, **47**: 4248–4253.

20 Stanton, L.W., Schwab, M. and Bishop, J.M. Nucleotide sequence of the human N-myc gene. *Proc Natl Acad Sci USA*. 1986, **85**: 1772–1776.

21 Kaneko, Y., Kanda, N., Maseki, N. *et al*. Different karyotypic patterns in early and advanced stage neuroblastomas. *Cancer Res*. 1987, **47**: 311–318.

22 Ikegaki, N., Bugovsky, J. and Kennet, R.H. Identification and characterisation of the N-myc gene product in human neuroblastoma cells by monoclonal

antibodies with defined specificities. *Proc Natl Acad Sci USA.* 1986, **83**: 5929–5933.

23 Rijinders, A.W.M., Van der Korput, J.A.G.M., Van Steenbrugge, G.J. *et al.* Expression of cellular oncogenes in human prostatic carcinoma cell lines. *Biochem Biophys Res Commun.* 1985, **132**: 548–554.

24 Viola, M.V., Fromowitz, F., Oravez, F. *et al.* Expression of ras oncogene p21 in prostate cancer. *New Engl J Med.* 1986, **314**: 133–137.

25 Shapiro, J.R. Biology of gliomas: heterogeneity, oncogenes, growth factors. *Semin Oncol.* 1986, **13**: 4–15.

26 Seizinger, S., De la Monte, S., Atkins, L. *et al.* Molecular genetic approach to human meningioma: loss of genes on chromosome 22. *Proc Natl Acad Sci USA.* 1987, **84**: 5419–5423.

27 Garson, J.A., McIntyre, P.G. and Kemshead, J.T. N-myc amplification in malignant astrocytoma (letter). *Lancet.* 1985, **2**: 718–719.

28 Fujita, J., Yoshida, O., Yuasa, Y. *et al.* Ha-ras oncogenes are activated by somatic alterations in human urinary tract tumours. *Nature.* 1984, **309**: 464–466.

29 Malone, P.R., Visvanathan, K.V., Ponder, B.A.J. *et al.* Oncogenes and bladder cancer. *Br J Urol.* 1985, **57**: 664–667.

30 Fearon, E.R., Feinberg, A.P., Hamilton, S.H. and Vogelstein, B. Loss of genes on the short arm of chromosome 11 in bladder cancer. *Nature.* 1985, **318**: 377–380.

31 De Martinville, B., Giacalone, J., Shih, C. *et al.* Oncogene from human EJ bladder carcinoma is located on the short arm of chromosome 11. *Science.* 1983, **219**: 499–501.

32 McBride, O.W., Swan, D.C., Santos, E. *et al.* Localisation of the normal allele of T24 human bladder carcinoma oncogene to chromosome 11. *Nature.* 1982, **300**: 773–776.

33 Marshall, C.J., Vousden, K.H. and Phillips, D.H. Activation of c-H-ras-1 proto-oncogene by *in vitro* modification with a chemical carcinogen, benzo-alpha-pyrenediol-epoxide. *Nature.* 1984, **310**: 586–589.

34 Dubeau, L. and Jones, P.A. Growth of normal and neoplastic urothelium and response to epidermal growth factor in a defined serum-free medium. *Cancer Res.* 1987, **47**: 2107–2112.

35 Green, S., Walter, P., Kumar, V. *et al.* Human oestrogen receptor cDNA sequence, expression and homology to v-erb-A. *Nature.* 1986, **320**: 134–139.

36 Law, M.L., Kao, F.T., Wei, Q. *et al.* The progesterone receptor gene maps to human chromosome band 11q13, the site of the mammary oncogene int-2. *Proc Natl Acad Sci USA.* 1986, **84**: 2877–2881.

37 Sainsbury, J.R.C., Farndon, J.R., Sherbet, G.V. and Harris, A.L. Epidermal growth factor receptors and oestrogen receptors in human breast cancer. *Lancet.* 1985, **1**: 364–366.

38 Kasid, A., Lippman, M.E., Papageorge, A.G. *et al.* Transfection of v-ras DNA into MCF-7 human breast cells bypasses dependence on oestrogen for tumourigenicity. *Science.* 1985, **228**: 725–728.

39 Theillet, C., Lidereau, R., Escot, C. *et al.* Loss of a c-H-ras-1 allele and aggressive human primary breast carcinomas. *Cancer Res.* 1986, **46**: 4776–4781.

40 Horan Hand, P., Vilasi, V., Thor, A., Ohuchi, N. and Schlom, J. Quantitation of Harvey ras p21 enhanced expression in human breast and colon carcinomas. *JNCI.* 1987, **79**: 59–65.

41 Escot, C., Theillet, R., Lidereau, R. *et al.* Genetic alteration of the c-myc proto-oncogene (MYC) in human primary breast carcinomas. *Proc Natl Acad Sci USA.* 1986, **83**: 4834–4838.

42 Huff, K.K., Kaufman, D., Gabbay, K.H. *et al.* Secretion of an insulin-like growth

factor-1 related protein by human breast cancer cells. *Cancer Res*. 1986, **46**: 4613–4619.

43 Brozert, D.A., Pantazis, P., Antoniades, H.N. *et al*. Synthesis and secretion of platelet-derived growth factor by human breast cancer cell lines. *Proc Natl Acad Sci USA*. **84**: 5763–5767.

44 Sainsbury, J.R.C., Farndon, J.R., Needham, G.K. *et al*. Epidermal growth factor receptor status as predictor of early recurrence of and death from breast cancer. *Lancet*. 1987. **38**: 1398–1402.

45 Kudlow, J.E., Cheung, C-Y.M. and Bjorge, J.D. Epidermal growth factor stimulates the synthesis of its own receptor in a human breast cancer cell line. *J Biol Chem*. 1986, **261**: 4134–4138.

2 ONCOPROTEINS AND THEIR FUNCTION IN THE TRANSFORMED CELL

J.V. WATSON AND K. SIKORA

THERE ARE three conventional approaches to the treatment of cancer, surgery, radiotherapy and chemotherapy. Surgery and radiotherapy are effective in dealing with local disease in a wide variety of malignancies. In metastatic cancer, chemotherapy is only effective in prolonging survival in certain relatively rare tumour types. The problem in disseminated malignancy in devising strategies for selective tumour cell destruction is the similarity of the cancer cell to its normal counterpart.

Oncogenes are a family of unique sequences of DNA whose abnormal expression is associated with the development of malignant transformation. The exact mechanisms by which malignant transformation is achieved remain unclear, but sequence homology between oncoproteins, the peptide products of oncogenes and growth factors and their receptors, together with functional characteristics that point to a role for these products in cell cycle control, provide intriguing leads in the study of the signalling mechanisms that regulate cell growth. When activated by the process of amplification, mutation, translocation and deletion, genes can promote tumour formation by means of their products. Recent techniques in oligopeptide immunisation have been used to develop sets of monoclonal antibodies against oncogene products. These novel reagents have been used to investigate oncogene function in normal and neoplastic tissue and have already demonstrated their potential as tumour markers with prognostic capability for purifying and analysing oncoproteins. Their function can also be explored and may open new avenues for specific therapy. In this chapter current developments in this field are reviewed.

The first connection between oncoproteins and proliferation control was made in 1983 when c-sis was shown to encode a subunit of platelet derived growth factor, PDGF, [1, 2]. This association was consolidated in the succeeding two years when the v-erbB and c-fms genes respectively were shown to encode the intracellular domain of the receptor for epidermal growth factor, EGF, [3] and a transmembrane receptor for macrophage colony stimulating factor, CSF1 [4, 5].

21

However, disordered proliferation control is only one aspect of cancer. The second major characteristic is the propensity for metastasis. Further discoveries have potentially linked this phenomenon with disordered functioning of oncogenes encoding cytoskeleton elements. The v-*fgr* gene encodes a hybrid protein containing a portion of the actin molecule [6] and *onc*-D codes for a non-muscle tropomyosin [7].

ONCOPROTEIN FUNCTION

Although specific biochemical functions have been assigned to some of the oncoproteins [8] we do not, as yet, know how alterations of these can lead to the neoplastic phenotype. Duesberg, playing devil's advocate, has pointed out that the only 'true' oncogenes are those found in retroviruses [9]. These genes have the capacity not only to induce, but also to maintain malignant transformation apparently in a single step by either insertion of a gene, or a long terminal repeat acting as a promotor or both. The protein products of c-*sis*, c-*erbB* and c-*fms* are undoubtedly concerned with growth control. The virally encoded proteins almost certainly mimic their cellular counterparts, but allow the cell to change gear in growth potential. The viral on-cogene products are related at least in part to their cellular homologues [10]. Apart from that, our detailed knowledge of oncoprotein function and the physiology which underlies transformation is scanty. Further-more, the oncogenes to be found in retroviruses are not precisely identical to their cellular homologues, the proto-oncogenes [11]. As a result of the molecular pathology induced by carcinogenesis, either the coding or control regions of the proto-oncogenes are modified [12, 13]. These changes can subvert the normal growth control proces-ses by increased, or inappropriate, production of normal oncogene products, or by expression of aberrant proteins [14, 15]. However, although our lack of physiological understanding is enormous, these are very interesting observations which will eventually form into a coherent whole. Part of the problem in our understanding the function of both cellular and viral oncoproteins, is that most of our information about them has come through molecular genetics. Thus, whilst there is a plethora of data on sequences, intron–exon structure and chromosomal location our knowledge of the proteins themselves has so far been scant.

The v-*sis* protein can transform appropriate cells but PDGF cannot. However, v-*sis* encodes only the B subunit of the growth factor. The product of either v-*sis* or its cellular homologue may not have to be secreted from the cell to produce transformation [16]. Hence, inappropriately increased production of the B subunit may 'short-circuit' one of the normal proliferation control mechanisms within the cell. The normal c-*fos* protein does not induce transformation, but modification of the carboxy terminus by manipulation of the gene can give rise to transformation [17]. There is also a difference between the carboxy termini of p60 v-*src* and p60 c-*src* which may be related to the transforming capacity of the former [18].

CYTOPLASMIC ONCOPROTEINS

Many of these proteins, including those encoded by *erb*B, *fms*, *yes*, *src*, *ras*, *mos* and *fes* to mention but a few, have protein kinase activity [19]. P60 v-*src* phosphorylates tyrosine [20] and is found in adhesion plaques of infected cells [21]. These findings have aroused interest as tyrosine is one of the more unusual amino acids to undergo phosphorylation and the cytoskeleton protein vinculin is abundant in adhesion plaques. It anchors actin mcrofilaments to the plasma membrane which is part of the mechanism responsible for adherence of cells to the substratum. The tyrosine residues of vinculin are specifically hyperphosphorylated by a factor of about eight in Rous sarcoma virus infected cells compared with uninfected cells [22]. This modifies the protein's normal function. Cells infected with heat sensitive Rous sarcoma virus mutants [23] exhibit dramatic cytoskeleton changes at p60 v-*src* permissive temperatures. Within 15–20 minutes of a temperature decrease, 'flowers' observed by fluorescence, appeared on the upper surface of infected cells. These 'flowers' are composed of myosin, tropomyosin, and actin [24] and it is postulated that a microfilament-anchorage protein, as yet unidentified, might serve as a direct target for p60 v-*src*. This may well be vinculin.

Another major set of cytoplasmic oncogene products are those coded for by the *ras* gene family. Three members have been identified so far, Ki-*ras*, Ha-*ras* and N-*ras*. The molecular weight of their encoded protein is 21 000. The protein remains in the cytoplasm although in some cases it is associated relatively loosely with the cell membrane. Related proteins have been identified in yeast and are thought to be involved in a signal transmission [25]. One common feature of the *ras* gene oncoproteins is their capability to bind GTP. They also have intrinsic GTPase activity cleaving GTP into GDP, controlling intracellular pool levels of a variety of nuclear tri- and diphosphates. The exact mechanism of action of p21 N-*ras* is unclear. A product of the N-*ras* gene p21 N-*ras* seems to link the effects of growth factor stimulation of receptors with inositol phospholipid metabolism [26] which is increased in cells stimulated into the division cycle. Increased phosphoinositol turnover is mediated via a guanine nucleotide regulatory G-protein which may, therefore, be p21 N-*ras* or a closely related species.

Altered forms of *ras* genes have been implicated in transfection assays. In 1982, two independent groups demonstrated clearly that the transforming sequence from a human bladder carcinoma was indeed a modified form of H-*ras*. The p21 protein able to transfect was found to have a point mutation at position 12, which results in the substitution of a glycine by valine. A variety of other point mutations have now been identified in the *ras* gene which results in positive transfection assays using a variety of recipient cell lines. These cluster around position 12 and 61. More recently, intriguing studies using site directed mutagenesis have attempted to evaluate the role of GTP binding with *ras* gene function [27]. The contact site for the guanine component of GTP is an asparagine in position 116. When this is changed to glutamine GTP binding affinity is reduced 10%. When isoleucine is substituted there is no GTP binding. A variety of *ras* constructs containing mutations at various positions were used to transfect a recipient cell line in a transfection model. Those constructs unable to bind GTP or showing reduced binding were still able to transform the cell. Therefore, transformation ability and GTP binding does not necessarily correlate completely.

P53 has been implicated not only in transformation [28, 29] but also in cell proliferation [30, 31, 32, 33]. Elevated levels are found in cells transformed by radiation and chemicals as well as with viral agents [34, 35, 36, 37, 38]. This oncoprotein may play a part in regulation of DNA synthesis as microinjection of an anti-p53 monoclonal antibody inhibits growth factor induced DNA synthesis in 3T3 cells [39]. However, p53 is a normal protein functioning in proliferation control [30, 31, 40]. We can surmise that expression of p53 must be under extremely strict regulation in normal cells in order to contain its oncogenic potential. This control can operate at several levels including transcription [30], mRNA transcript copy number [41] and protein turnover [40, 42]. It also appears to exist in two distinct forms. A number of antibodies have been raised to this protein and Milner [43] has shown that one antibody recognises a p53 epitope in quiescent cells which is occluded after stimulation. A second antibody recognises an epitope after stimulation which is not exposed before stimulation. Both antibodies immunoprecipitate at 53 kd. These results suggest that there may be a conformational change in the protein after stimulation which is related to the different functional states of quiescent and stimulated cells.

NUCLEAR ONCOPROTEINS

At least three cellular oncogenes with viral homologues (*fos*, *myb* and *myc*) encode proteins which are nuclear associated. The functions of these proteins are not yet known although increasing evidence suggests that the c-*myc* product is involved in cell proliferation regulation [44, 45, 46, 47, 48]. It may also play a part in differentiation as mRNA copy number shows a peak at 4–5 weeks in developing placenta [49] and a peak during spermatogenesis with germ cells and mature sperm showing very low levels [50]. This protein has a molecular weight of 62 kd, p62 c-*myc*, and is one of a discrete set of non-histone and non-matrix nuclear proteins which elute from the nucleus at salt concentrations below 200 mmol [51]. This suggests a nuclear binding function which can be modulated rapidly by ionic changes within the physiological range. The turnover of both the protein and its mRNA are rapid with half-lives in the order 20–30 minutes in exponentially growing cells [52]. C-myc mRNA exhibited an increase within two hours of serum stimulation in serum deprived cells but did not, thereafter, show a cyclical variation correlating with cell cycle phase or decrease in density arrested cells maintained in the presence of growth factors [53]. The most recent evidence suggest that p62 c-*myc* is intimately involved in the replication complex of proteins responsible for the initiation and maintenance of DNA synthesis [54].

PROLIFERATION CONTROL

Although detailed information is still sparse, it is quite obvious that oncogenes encode proteins which are intimately involved in the basic control mechanisms of one of the most fundamental of all cellular functions, the drive to proliferate. Normally, growth is tightly regulated with considerable precision by a well integrated molecular chain carrying signals from the exterior to the nucleus. The available evidence suggests that there will be a number of sub-categories, at least five, involved in proliferation. These include genes encoding extracellular signal transmitters (c-sis), signal receivers on the external membrane (c-fms), intracellular transmitters (c-ras) and signal receivers and transducers in the nucleus. Likely possibilities for the last category include the oestrogen receptor, which has recently been shown to have extensive homology with the steroid receptor encoded by v-erbA oncogene [55], and the proteins encoded by c-myc, c-fos and c-myb. There is some evidence already that p62 c-myc is concerned with triggering or maintaining stimulated cells in division. P53 is also a candidate with a possible role in the initiation and/or control of DNA synthesis.

It would seem possible that growth factors such as EGF and possibly also transferrin, the interleukins and insulin together with their receptors will be found to be encoded by oncogenes. It is becoming increasingly obvious that these genes are not exclusive to cancer, rather that they first became apparent in cancer through the virus connection and their involvement in proliferation. All diseases in which proliferation or differentiation are disordered or required, including, for example, both rheumatoid and osteo-arthritis, granulomatous processes, proliferative vasculitis, bone marrow response to anaemia or infection and wound healing are likely to be accompanied by alterations in oncogene expression.

Some aspects of the cancer jig-saw which relate to proliferation are beginning to fall into place. However, we have hardly begun to address the most important aspect of human cancer in practical terms, that of metastasis. The majority of unsuccessfully treated cancer patients die from metastatic disease as local disease is generally curable. In cancer inappropriate cell proliferation is most likely to be due to failure of negative servocontrol mechanisms which normally regulate growth to within extraordinarily narrow limits. By the same token, the metastasis phenomenon is also likely to be due to a failure of control mechanisms which would normally constrain cells to recognise their correct 'geographical' location. All cells possess the potential capacity for mobility. Metastatic cancer cells exhibit inappropriate mobility. Mobility is associated with motility and the proteins of the cytoskeleton confer motility. It would seem to be highly significant that two oncogenes, v-fgr and onc-D, encode cytoskeleton elements both coupled with tyrosine kinase activity [6, 7]. Thus, we have a second major category of 'oncogenes', those concerned with sub-cellular architecture and hence possibly with metastatic potential, to complement disordered proliferation and metastasis.

RELEVANCE OF ONCOGENES TO HUMAN CANCER

Clinical observation does not support a single step to the malignant phenotype as observed with retroviruses in animals. Hyperkeratotic lesions of the hands and face of Caucasians exposed to tropical sun may or may not progress to frankly invasive squamous cell carcinoma. Few would doubt that the lesions are premalignant. Villous adenomas of the colon are recognised as being premalignant but the final transformation to the fully malignant invasive phenotype may take years. Another good example is transitional cell papillomas of the bladder which may take 20 years before invasion takes place. Also, the bladder lining may undergo metaplastic change to a squamous epithelium in response to the chronic irritation of vesicolithiasis before the development of squamous cancer. Carcinoma *in situ* of the uterine cervix may considerably antedate invasion of the basement membrane as may comparable ductal epithelial changes in the breast. A loose parallel has been found in model systems. Land, Parada and Weinberg have shown that full transformation to a neoplastic phenotype may require the 'co-operation' of two or more genes [56]. A *ras* gene point mutation did not transform, but combined co-transfection with v-*myc* gave rise to full transformation. A similar phenomenon was also found with p53 and *ras* [57].

The vast majority of studies carried out to date in both tissue culture and in human cancer have relied upon hybridization techniques using radioactive probes for either DNA [58] or mRNA [59]. These methods, particularly the latter, require fresh tissue which is not always obtainable in sufficient quantities from cancer patients. Also, it may take a considerable time to accumulate sufficient material and information to make meaningful clinical correlates with fresh tissue. This applies particularly to the rare tumours. Pathological departments are notorious for hoarding their archival material which contains a huge store of information locked up in wax awaiting release. Moreover, neither the gene nor its message is the effector molecule; this is the province of the protein. Herein lie the possibilities for extending clinical applications using monoclonal antibodies directed to specific oncoproteins, for example p53 [60], p21 c-*ras* [61] and p62 c-*myc* [62]. Antibodies can now be raised to hydrophillic synthetic peptides predicted from the base sequence of cloned genes. As many oncogenes have now been completely sequenced, panels of such antibodies are being used for routine use in diagnosis, screening, monitoring, prognosis and some may have possible therapeutic application. A variety of such antibodies are already commercially available for research purposes (Table 2.1).

Table 2.1 Antibodies currently available to oncogene products

Oncoprotein	Antibody	Immunohistology	Manufacturer
pan *myc*	Sheep PCA	+	CRB
c-*myc*	Sheep PCA	+	CRB
	Mouse MCA	+	CRB
	Sheep PCA	+	BIOTX
	Sheep PCA	?	ONCOR
N-*myc*	Sheep PCA	+	CRB
L-*myc*	Sheep PCA	?	CRB
K-*ras*	Mouse MCA	+	CETUS
N-*ras*	Mouse MCA	+	CETUS
H-*ras*	Mouse MCA	+	CETUS
	Sheep PCA	+	BIOTX
	Sheep PCA	?	ONCOR
c-*ras*	Mouse MCA	+	CETUS
	Sheep PCA	?	BIOTX
c-*ras* ser12	Mouse MCA	?	CETUS
c-*ras* val12	Mouse MCA	?	CETUS
c-*ras* arg12	Mouse MCA	?	CETUS
c-*ras* asp12	Mouse MCA	?	CETUS
pan-*fos*	Sheep PCA	+	CRB
c-*fos*	Sheep PCA	+	CRB
	Sheep PCA	+	BIOTX
c-*src*	Mouse MCA	?	ONCOR
c-*myb*	Sheep PCA	?	CRB
c-*fms*	Rabbit PCA	?	CRB
c-*mos*	Rabbit PCA	?	CRB
c-*erb*B1	Mouse MCA	?	AMERSHAM
c-*erb*B1	Mouse MCA	?	ONCOR
c-*erb*B1	Rabbit PCA	+	CRB

ANTI-ONCOPROTEIN ANTIBODIES: FUTURE APPLICATIONS

Anti-oncoprotein antibodies have now been used for localisation in tissue sections and for quantitation of levels in serum, urine and in populations of single cells.

Diagnosis, screening, prognosis and monitoring

Immunocytochemical localisation with antibodies has been used to define differential ras expression in benign and malignant colonic disease [63]. Studies with an anti-p62 c-*myc* monoclonal antibody, MYC 1-6E10 [62], have shown that normal colonic mucosa exhibited maximal expression in the maturation zones of the crypts of Lieber-kuhn where there was mixed nuclear and cytoplasmic staining [64]. However, p62 c-*myc* is known to be nuclear associated and in further more extensive studies it has been shown that this protein is redistributed from a nuclear to a cytoplasmic location with increasing maturation of the normal colonic mucosa [65]. This has also been shown in mucosa freshly fixed within seconds of biopsy [66]. Active exclusion of the protein from the nucleus may be part of the normal control mechanism for regulating proliferation and differentiation. In familial polyposis coli, which inexorably progresses to the malignant invasive phenotype, nuclear staining persisted to the surface of the crypts and in carcinomas the staining is predominantly nuclear [65]. Quantitative studies comparing normal with dysplastic mucosa and carcinomas developing in patients with ulcerative colitis have shown that the nuclear p62 c-*myc* content increased with the transition from 'mild' to 'severe' dysplasia [66] and that the protein content is raised in carcinomas [67]. Furthermore, the protein content was also raised in morphologically normal colonic mucosa derived from malignant compared with non-malignant specimens [68]. These studies used flow cytometric techniques [69, 70, 71] to quantitate the oncoprotein content with total DNA simultaneously in individual nuclei extracted from tissue sections [72] using an adaptation of the method of Hedley *et al.* [73]. The results from archival material using fluorescence techniques complemented those obtained with Northern and Western blotting using fresh tissue [74].

Studies have also been carried out in testicular cancer biopsies. p62 c-*myc* was expressed in only small amounts in the normal testis. Seminomas exhibited increased nuclear and cytoplasmic staining. Undifferentiated teratomas showed barely detectable staining whereas well differentiated epithelial structures and yolk-sac elements exhibited intense staining [75]. Parallel flow cytometric quantitation was carried out which enabled significant limits to be assigned to the qualitative results obtained by immunocytochemistry. Low p62 c-*myc* levels were found in normal testicular tissue and significantly elevated levels were found from teratoma [$p<0.001$) and seminoma ($p<0.001$). However, the oncoprotein level increased significantly with increasing differentiation in teratoma ($p<0.01$). Patients with intermediate and undifferentiated tumours who developed recurrence had lower levels than those who remained disease free, ($p<0.05$) [76] hence prognostic information is potentially forthcoming. Sainsbury *et al.* [77] have also obtained prognostic information in breast cancer patients by assaying EGF receptor (v-*erb*B) and oestrogen receptor (v-*erb*A).

Flow technology has been used in uterine cervix neoplasia to assay for p62 c-*myc* in archival specimens [78]. Normal biopsies exhibited higher p62 c-*myc* levels than carcinomas ($p<0.00001$). There was a progressive decrease in oncoprotein level with progression from cervical intraepithelial neoplasia, stage I (CIN I) to CIN III ($p<0.05$). Furthermore, the maximum fluorescence signal in the normal tissues occurred at a lower antibody concentration compared with tumour tissue ($p<0.01$). There was no correlation with histological grade, stage, age or prognosis in patients with invasion. These techniques have now been adapted for tissue sampled from colposcopy clinics with a view to automated prescreening of cervical smears in an attempt to exploit the obvious diagnostic potential of the simultaneous DNA/ p62 c-*myc* assay [79].

The findings in colonic neoplasia and seminoma were partially anticipated but those in both the histological breakdown of teratoma and in cervical carcinoma were completely contrary to expectation. The latter finding was particularly controversial as Riou *et al.* [80] have reported amplification of both the c-*myc* and H-*ras* oncogenes in carcinoma of the cervix associated with papilloma virus infection. However, an increase in either the gene or mRNA copy number, which should give rise to an increased protein production rate, need not necessarily be reflected in a marked increase in the total protein content for two main reasons. Firstly, inappropriately increased message may result in rate limitation at the protein synthesis level. Secondly, an increase in protein degradation may offset an increased production rate. The latter is most likely to occur with a protein which has a short half-life and clearly, this is a distinct possibility for p62 c-*myc* with a half life of 20–30 minutes in rapidly cycling and stimulated cells [47, 48]. The lower absolute levels in carcinoma of the cervix compared with normal cervix, and in the undifferentiated compared with the better differentiated teratomas, may reflect increased protein turnover and an increased cell production rate in the former. Further possibilities include post-translational protein modification in the more malignant teratomas and in cervical carcinoma giving rise to an alteration or partial occlusion of the epitope recognised by the antibody, and a possible increase in the susceptibility of the protein to proteolysis in neoplastic cells as a result of the assay procedure itself. There is some evidence that post-translational protein modification may occur in cervical carcinoma. Maximum binding was observed at different antibody concentrations in the normal and malignant cells which might indicate a change in binding constant.

These various findings suggest a potential for the oncoproteins to become a new generation of tumour markers, and in this context it is significant that they have also been detected in serum and urine. Antibodies against the cellular protein p53 have been detected in sera from patients with breast cancer [81]. Anti-peptide antibodies have detected and compared oncogene-related proteins in urine in normal subjects, pregnant women and in cancer patients. Similar studies have been conducted using an antibody to the c-*myc* protein. A 40 000 molecular weight breakdown product of p62 c-*myc*, or a related protein, was detected in cancer patients and in pregnancy [82] and the p40 serum levels decreased after hemi-colectomy for carcinomas, raising the possibility of monitoring for recurrence by regular sampling. Diagnostic scanning is another possibility as a radiolabelled anti-p62 c-*myc* antibody has been used to localise lung cancer [83].

Therapy

The scope for developing diagnostic, screening, prognostic and monitoring assays using probes for the oncogenes and their products is enormous. Although it is clear how these assays might relate to overall patient management, it is not so obvious how a knowledge of oncogenes and their products will relate directly to therapy. Nevertheless, possibilities do exist. Tamoxifen has been used for breast cancer patients for almost two decades, yet it is only recently that oestrogen receptor has been shown to be homologous with part of the protein encoded by v-*erb*A [84]. Moreover, many of the oncoproteins involved in pathological processes are slightly abnormal; examples from experimental systems include those encoded by *fos* and *src*. The v-*erb*B oncogene encodes the intracellular and transmembrane domains plus a truncated portion of the external domain of the EGF receptor in some human cancers. If this truncated extracellular domain is unique to the tumour cells in which it is found it may be possible to use specified monoclonal antibody mediated cell-killing with coupled toxins or radioisotopes. Complement mediated killing is another possibility.

CONCLUSIONS

It is unlikely that all oncoproteins will be found to be abnormal in human cancer. However, if any intracellular oncoproteins are found to be abnormal they could be blocked by small synthetic peptides without blocking the normal counterpart. These possibilities are mere speculation at present and it seems highly unlikely that a universal 'oncogene-related magic bullet' will be forthcoming for all cancer. Full therapeutic possibilities will have to await the complete elucidation of oncogene physiology. However, a real start has been made and we believe that we are just at the very beginning of a renaissance in cancer treatment which will be based on an understanding of the fundamental biochemical differences between normal and malignant cells. That understanding will come from objective measurements made at the molecular level and the differences will be exploited for the benefit of the cancer patient.

REFERENCES

1 Doolittle, R.F., Hunkerpiller, M.W., Hood, L.E., Devare, S.G., Robbins, K.C., Aaronson, S.A. and Antoniades, H.W. Simian sarcoma virus onc gene, v-sis, is derived from the gene (or genes) encoding a platelet derived growth factor. *Science*. 1983, **211**: 275–276.

2 Waterfield, M.D., Scrace, G.T., Whittle, N. *et al*. Platelet derived growth factor is structurally related to the putative transforming protein p^{28sis} of simian sarcoma virus. *Nature*. 1983, **304**: 35–39.

3 Downward, J., Yardem, Y., Mayes, E. *et al*. Close similarities of epidermal growth factor receptor and v-erbB oncogene. *Nature*. 1984, **307**: 521–527.

4 Roussel, M.F., Rettenmier, C.W., Look, A.T. and Scherr, C.J. Cell surface expression of v-fms-coded glycoproteins is required for transformation. *Mol Cell Biol*. 1984, **4**: 1999–2009.

5 Scherr, C.J., Rettenmier, C.W., Sacca, R., Roussel, M.F., Look, A.T. and Stanley, E.R. The c-fms proto-oncogene product is related to the receptor for the mononuclear phagocytic growth factor, CSF 1. *Cell*. 1985, **41**: 665–676.

6 Naharro, G., Robins, K. and Reddy, E.P. Gene product of v-fgr onc: hybrid protein contains a portion of actin and a tyrosine-specific protein kinase. *Science*. 1984, **223**: 63–66.

7 Martin-Zanca, D., Hughes, S.H. and Barbacid, M. A human oncogene formed by the fusion of truncated tropomyosin and protein tyrosine kinase sequences. *Nature.* 1986, **319**: 743–748.

8 Bishop, J.M. Trends in oncogenes. *Trends Genet.* 1984, **1**: 245–249.

9 Duesberg, P.H. Activated proto-onc genes: sufficient or necessary for cancer? *Science.* 1985, **228**: 660–677.

10 Schechter, A.L., Stern, D.F., Vaidyanathan, V., Decker, S. J., Drebin, J.A., Green, M.I. and Weinberg, R.A. The neu oncogene: an erb-B-related gene encoding a 185,000-M_t tumour antigen. *Nature.* 1984, **312**: 513–517.

11 Hunter, T. Oncogenes and proto-oncogenes: how do they differ? *J Natl Cancer Inst.* 1984, **73**: 773–785.

12 Cooper, G.M. and Lane, M.A. Cellular transforming genes and oncogenesis. *Biochim Biophys Acta.* 1984, **738**: 9–20.

13 Krontiris, T.G. The emerging genetics of human cancer. *New Eng J Med.* 1983, **309**: 404–409.

14 Der, C.J. and Cooper, G.M. Altered gene products are associated with activation of cellular ras^K genes in human lung and colon carcinomas. *Cell.* 1983; **32**: 201–208.

15 Stewart, T.A., Pattengale, P.K. and Leder, P. Spontaneous mammary adenocarcinomas in transgenic mice carry and express MTV/myc fusion genes. *Cell.* 1984, **38**: 627–637.

16 Betsholtz, C., Wetermark, B., Ek, B. and Heidin, C.H. Coexpression of a PDGF-like growth factor and PDGF receptors in a human osteosarcoma cell line: implications for autocrine receptor activation. *Cell.* 1984, **39**: 447–457.

17 Miller, A.D., Curran, T. and Verma, I.M. C-fos protein can induce cellular transformation: a novel mechanism for activation of a cellular oncogene. *Cell.* 1984, **36**: 51–60.

18 Takeya, H. and Hanafusa, H. Structure and sequence of the cellular gene homologous to the RSV src gene and the mechanism for generating the transforming virus. *Cell.* 1983, **32**: 881–890.

19 Hunter, T. and Cooper, J.A. Protein-tyrosine kinases. *Annu Rev Biochem.* 1985, **54**: 897–930.

20 Hunter, T. and Sefton, B.M. Transforming gene product of Rous sarcoma virus phosphorylates tyrosine. *Proc Natl Acad Sci USA.* 1980, **77**: 1311–1315.

21 Rohrschneider, L.R. Adhesion plaques of Rous sarcoma virus transformed cells contain the src gene product. *Proc Natl Acad Sci USA.* 1980, **77**: 3514–3518.

22 Sefton, B.M., Hunter, T., Ball, E.H. and Singer, S.J. Vinculin: a cytoskeletal target for the transforming protein of Rous sarcoma virus. *Cell.* 1981, **24**: 165–174.

23 Martin, G.S. Rous sarcoma virus; a function required for the maintenance of the transformed state. *Nature.* 1970, **227**: 1021–1023.

24 Boschek, C.B., Jockusch, B.M., Friis, R.R., Back, R., Grundmann, E. and Bauer, H. Early changes in the distribution and organisation of microfilament proteins during cell transformation. *Cell.* 1981, **24**: 175–184.

25 Hurley, J.B., Simon, M.I., Teplow, D.B., Robinshaw, J.D. and Gilman, A.G. Homologies between signal transducing G proteins and ras gene products. *Science.* 1984, **226**: 860–863.

26 Wakelman, M.J.O., Davies, S.A., Houslay, M.D., McKay, I., Marshall, C.J. and Hall, A. Normal $p^{21N\text{-}ras}$ couples bombesin and other growth factors to inositole phosphate production. *Nature*. 1986, **323**: 173–176.

27 McCormick, F., Clark, B.F., La Cour, R.F., Kjeldgaard, M., Nybore, J. A model for the territory structure of p21—the product of the ras oncogene. *Science*. 1985, **230**: 78–82.

28 Crawford, L.V., Pim, D.C. and Bulbrook, R.D. Detection of antibodies against the cellular protein p^{53} in sera from patients with breast cancer. *Int J Cancer*. 1982, **30**: 403–408.

29 Eliyahu, D., Raz, A., Gruss, P., Gival, D. and Oren, M. Participation of p^{53} cellular tumour antigen in transformation of normal embryonal cells. *Nature*. 1984, **312**: 646–649.

30 Mercer, W.E., Nelson, D., Deleo, A.B., Old, L.J. and Baserga. R. Microinjection of monoclonal antibody to protein p^{53} inhibits serum-induced DNA synthesis in 3T3 cells. *Proc Natl Acad Sci USA*. 1982, **79**: 6309–6312.

31 Milner, J. and McCormick, F. Lymphocyte stimulation: concanavalin A induces the expression of a 53K protein. *Cell Biol Int Rep*. 1980, **4**: 663–667.

32 Milner, J. and Milner, S. SV40-53K antigen: a possible role for 53K in normal cells. *Virology*. 1981, **112**: 785–788.

33 Sarnow, P., Ho, Y.S., Williams, J. and Levine, A.J. Adenovirus Elb-58K tumour antigen and SV40 large tumour antigen are physically associated with the same 54kd cellular protein in transformed cells. *Cell*. 1981, **28**: 387–394.

34 Deleo, A.B., Jay, G., Appella, E., Dubois, G.C., Law, L.W. and Old, J. Detection of a transformation-related antigen in chemically induced sarcomas and other transformed cells in the mouse. *Proc Natl Acad Sci USA* 1979, **76**: 2420–2424.

35 Lane, D.P. and Crawford, L.V. T-antigen is bound to a host protein in SV40-transformed cells. *Nature*. 1979, **278**: 261–602.

36 Linzer, D.I.H. and Levine, A.J. Characterisation of a 54k Dalton cellular SV40 tumour antigen present in SV40-transformed cells and uninfected embryonal carcinoma cells. *Cell*. 1979, **17**: 43–52.

37 Rotter, V. P^{53}, a transformation-related cellular-encoded protein, can be used as a biochemical marker for the detection of primary mouse tumour cells. *Proc Natl Acad Sci USA*. 1983, **80**: 2613–2617.

38 Boss, M.A., Dreyfuss, G and Baltimore, D. Localisation of the Abelson murine leukaemia virus protein in a detergent insoluble subcellular matrix. *J Virol*. 1981, **40**: 472–481.

39 Mercer, W.E., Nelson, D., Deleo, A.B., Old, L.J. and Baserga, R. Microinjection of monoclonal antibody to protein p^{53} inhibits serum-induced DNA synthesis in 3T3 cells. *Proc Natl Acad Sci USA*. 1982, **79**: 6309–6312.

40 Reich, N.C. and Levine, A.J. Growth regulation of a cellular tumour antigen, p^{53}, in non-transformed cells. *Nature*. 1984, **308**: 199–201.

41 Reich, N.C., Oren, M. and Levine, A.J. Two distinct mechanisms regulate the level of a cellular tumour antigen, p^{53}. *Mol Cell Biol*. 1983, **3**: 2143–2150.

42 Oren, M., Malzman, W. and Levine, A.J. Post-transitional regulation of the 54k cellular tumour antigen in normal and transformed cells. *Mol Cell Biol*. 1981, **1**: 101–110.

43 Milner, J. Different forms of p^{53} detected by monoclonal antibodies in non-dividing and dividing lymphocytes. *Nature*. 1984, **310**: 143–145.

44 Kelly, K., Cochran, B.H., Stiles, C.D. and Leder, P. Cell specific regulation of the c-myc gene by lymphocyte mitogens and platelet derived growth factor. 1983, **35**: 603–610.

45 Kelly, K., Cochran, B.H., Stiles, C.D. and Leder, P. The regulation of c-myc by growth signals. *Curr Topics Microbiol Immun*. 1984, **113**: 117–126.

46 Makino, R., Hayashi, K.A.and Sugimura, T. C-myc is induced in rat liver at a very early stage of regeneration or by cycloheximide treatment. *Nature*. 1984, **310**: 697–698.

47 Greenberg, M.E. and Ziff, E.B. Stimulation of 3T3 cells induces transcription of the c-fos proto-oncogene. *Nature*. 1984, **311**: 433–438.

48 Rabbitts, P.H., Watson, J.V., Lamond, A. *et al*. Metabolism of c-myc gene products: c-myc mRNA and protein expression in the cell cycle. *EMBO J*. 1985, **4**: 2009–2015.

49 Pfeiffer-Ohlsson, S., Goustin, A.S., Rydnert, J., Wahlstron, T., Bjersing, L., Stehelin, D. and Ohlsson, R. Spatial and temporal pattern of cellular myc oncogene expression in developing human placenta: implications for embryonic cell proliferation. *Cell*. 1984, **38**: 585–596.

50 Stewart, T.A., Bellve, A.R. and Leder, P. Transcription and promoter usage of the c-myc gene in normal somatic and spermatogenic cells. *Science*. 1984, **226**: 707–710.

51 Evan, G.I. and Hancock, D.C. Studies on the interaction of the human c-myc protein with cell nuclei: $p^{62c\text{-}myc}$ as a member of a discrete subset of nuclear proteins. *Cell*. 1985, **43**: 253–261.

52 Hann, S.R., Thompson, C.B. and Eisermann, R.N. C-myc oncogene protein is independent of the cell cycle in human and avian cells. *Nature*. 1985, **314**: 366–369.

53 Thompson, C.B., Challoner, P.B., Neiman, P.E. and Groudine, M. Levels of c-myc oncogene mRNA are invariate throughout the cell cycle. *Nature*. 1985, **314**: 363–366.

54 Studzinski, G.P., Brelvi, Z.S., Feldman, S.C. and Watt, R.A. Participation of c-myc in DNA synthesis of human cells. *Science*. 1986, **234**: 467–470.

55 Green, S., Walter, P., Kurman, V., Krust, A., Bornert, J.M., Argos, P. and Chambon, P. Human oestrogen receptor cDNA: sequence, expression and homology to v-erb-A. *Nature*. 1986, **320**: 134–139.

56 Land, H., Parada, L.F. and Weinberg, R.A. Tumourigenic conversion of primary embryo fibroblasts requires at least two cooperating oncogenes. *Nature*. 1983, **304**: 596–602.

57 Marx J. Cooperation between oncogenes. *Science*. 1983, **222**: 602–603.

58 Southern, E.M. Detection of specific sequences among DNA fragments by gel electrophoresis. *J Mol Biol*. 1975, **98**: 503–517.

59 Thomas, P.S. Hybridization of denatured RNA and small DNA fragments transferred to nitrocellulose. *Proc Natl Acad Sci USA*. 1980, **77**: 5201–5205.

60 Harlow, E., Crawford, L.V., Pim, P.C. and Williamson, N.M. Monoclonal antibodies specific for simian virus 40 tumour antigens. *J Virol*. 1981, **39**: 861–869.

61 Furth, M.E., Aldrich, T.H., Cordon-Cardo, C. Expression of ras proto-oncogene proteins in normal human tissues. *Oncogene*. 1987, **1**: 47–58.

62 Evan, G.I., Lewis, G.K., Ramsay, G. and Bishop, J.M. Isolation of monoclonal antibodies specific for human and mouse proto-oncogene products. *Mol Cell Biol*. 1985, **5**: 3160–3616.

63 Thor, A., Horan Hand, P., Wunderlich, D., Caruso, A., Muraro, R. and Schlom, J. Monoclonal antibodies define differential ras gene expression in malignant and benign colonic disease. *Nature*. 1984, **311**: 562–564.

64 Stewart, S.E., Evan, G.I., Watson, J.V. and Sikora, K.E. Detection of the c-myc oncogene product in colonic polyps and carcinomas. *Br J Cancer*. 1986, **53**: 1–6.

65 Sunderesan, V., Forgacs, I., Wight, D., Evan, G.I. and Watson, J.V. Abnormal distribution of the c-myc oncogene product in familial polyposis coli. *J Clin Pathol*. 1987, **40**: 1274–1281.

66 Forgacs, I.C., Sunderesan, V., Evan, G., Weight, D.G.D., Neale, G., Hunter, J.O. and Watson, J.V. Abnormal expression of c-myc oncogene product in dysplasia and neoplasia associated with ulcerative colitis. *Gut*. 1986, **7**: A1285.

67 Watson, J.V., Stewart, J., Cox, H., Sikora, K.E. and Evan, G.I. Flow cytometric quantitation of the c-myc oncoprotein in archival neoplastic biopsies of the colon. *Mol Cell Probes*. 1987, **1**: 151–157.

68 Watson, J.V., Stewart, J., Cox, H., Sikora, K.E. and Evan, G.I. c-myc onco-protein levels are raised in morphologically normal colonic mucosa derived from malignant compared with non-malignant specimens. (In submission.)

69 Watson, J.V. Enzyme kinetic studies in cell populations using fluorogenic substrates and flow cytometric techniques. *Cytometry*. 1980, **1**: 143–151.

70 Watson, J.V. Dual laser beam focussing for flow cytometry through a single crossed cylindrical lens pair. *Cytometry*. 1981, **2**: 14–19.

71 Watson, J.V. Flow cytometry in biomedical science. *Nature*, 1987, **325**: 741–742.

72 Watson, J.V., Sikora, K.E. and Evan, G.I. A simultaneous flow cytometric assay for c-myc oncoprotein and cellular DNA in nuclei from paraffin embedded material. *J Immunol Methods*. 1985, **83**: 179–192.

73 Hedley, D.W., Friedlander, M.I., Taylor, I.W., Rugg, C.A. and Musgrove, E.A. Method for analysis of cellular DNA content of paraffin-embedded pathological material using flow cytometry. *J Histochem Cytochem*. 1983, **31**: 1333–1335.

74 Sikora, K., Chan, S.Y.T., Evan, G.I., Markham, N., Stewart, J. and Watson, J.V. c-myc expression in colorectal cancer. *Cancer*. 1987b, **59**: 1289–1295.

75 Sikora, K., Evan, G., Stewart, J. and Watson, J.V. Detection of the c-myc oncogene product in testicular cancer. *Brit J Cancer*. 1985, **52**: 171–176.

76 Watson, J.V., Stewart, J., Evan, G., Ritson, A. and Sikora, K. The clinical significance of flow cytometric c-myc oncoprotein quantitation in testicular cancer. *Brit J Cancer*. 1986, **53**: 331–337.

77 Sainsbury, J.R.C., Farndon, J.R., Sherbet, G.V. and Harris, A.L. Epidermal growth factor receptors and oestrogen receptors in human breast cancer. *Lancet*. 1985, **i**: 364.

78 Hendy-Ibbs, P., Cox, H., Evan, G.I. and Watson, J.V. Flow cytometric quantitation of DNA and c-myc oncoprotein in archival biopsies of uterine cervix neoplasia. *Brit J Cancer*. 1987, **55**: 275–282.

79 Elias-Jones, J., Hendy-Ibbs, P., Cox, H., Evan, G.I. and Watson, J.V. Cervical brush biopsy specimens suitable for DNA and oncoprotein analysis using flow cytometry. *J Clin Pathol.* 1986, **39**: 577–581.

80 Riou, G., Barrois, M., Tordjman, I., Dutronquay, V. and Orth, G. Presence de genomes de papillomavirus et amplification des oncogenes c-myc et c-Ha-ras dans des cancers envahissants du col de l'uterus. *C R Soc Biol (Paris)* 1985, **299**: 575–580.

81 Crawford, L.V., Pim, D.C. and Bulbrook, R.D. Detection of antibodies against the cellular protein p^{53} in sera from patients with breast cancer. *Int J Cancer.* 1982, **30**: 403–408.

82 Sikora, K., Chan, S.Y.T., Evan, G.I., Gabri, H. and Hill, F. Detection of a p^{40} c-myc gene product-related protein in serum and urine of cancer patients. *Mol Cell Probes.* 1987a, **1**: 73–79.

83 Chan, S.Y.T., Evan, G.I., Ritson, A., Watson, J.V., Wright, P. and Sikora, K. Localisation of lung cancer by a radiolabelled monoclonal antibody against the c-myc oncogene product. *Brit J Cancer.* 1986, **54**: 761–769.

84 Green, S., Walter, P., Kurman, V., Krust, A., Bornert, J.M., Argos, P. and Chambon, P. Human oestrogen receptor cDNA: sequence, expression and homology to v-erb-A. *Nature.* 1986, **320**: 134–139.

3 THE C-*ERB*B2 GENE AND ITS EXPRESSION IN HUMAN TUMOURS

W.J. GULLICK AND D.J. VENTER

OVER THE last decade, about 40 genes have been described that have been implicated, directly or circumstantially, in the alteration of normal cells to immortalised or fully transformed cells. Most of these genes, called oncogenes, have been identified using two experimental systems. The first involves the analysis of acutely transforming animal retroviruses. These viruses have incorporated into their own structures host cellular genomic sequences. In many cases deletions and point mutations have occurred in the transduced sequence leading to the conversion of these normal, proto-oncogenes sequences into dominantly transforming viral oncogenes. Infection of animals with such viruses causes rapid and efficient tumourigenesis. Occasionally, cellular genes have been acquired by retroviruses that in themselves are not transforming oncogenes but provide assistance in the conversion of infected cells to a fully malignant phenotype. An example of such a gene is the v-*erb*A oncogene, recently shown to be related to the thyroid hormone receptor, which in itself is incapable of transforming cells, but in association with the v-*erb* gene, which encodes a fragment of the epidermal growth factor (EGF) receptor, potentiates the latter's ability to transform erythroblasts. The acquisition of more than one oncogene by a retrovirus, together with experiments demonstrating the co-operation of different classes of oncogenes in *in vitro* cell transformation is consistent with the multi-step models of carcinogenesis thought to occur *in vivo*.

The second system which has revealed genes as oncogenes is the transfection assay. Developed at the beginning of this decade, transfection involves isolating DNA from transformed cell lines or solid tumours and engendering its random uptake by immortalised but untransformed cells in culture. By this process, many cells acquire random DNA sequences but remain phenotypically normal. Occasionally, however, cells acquire transforming oncogenes derived from the tumour DNA whose expression in this new context leads to the uncontrolled growth of a clone of cells. These can be observed macroscopically and selected for further analysis. Oncogenes detected by transfection using the experimental systems currently employed are all therefore dominantly transforming. Several oncogenes encoded by retroviruses have also been detected by transfection, emphasising that perhaps relatively small numbers of cellular genes can be activated to dominant oncogenes. The transfection assay suffers from the drawback that cellular genes are often large, because of extensive intron sequences, and are technically difficult to transfect owing to fragmentation during isolation of the DNA. In fact, several oncogenes have been detected by this assay in which activating mutations have occurred due to recombination during the transfection procedure itself.

Much of this book concerns the nature of oncogenes and their products. This chapter concentrates on the c-erbB2 gene and protein which it encodes. This gene was originally detected by transfection but was subsequently shown to be structurally related to a retrovirally encoded oncogene, v-erbB.

RAT C-*NEU* AND *ONC-NEU* GENES

In the 1960s, a system of transplacental carcinogenesis was developed in which rodents were fed or injected with the chemical carcinogen, N-ethyl-N-nitrosourea (ENU). A single treatment of adult animals with ENU during late pregnancy by various systemic routes led to the frequent, almost inevitable, and selective occurrence of neoplasms in the central nervous system of the offspring. ENU decomposes rapidly *in vivo*, with a half life of 5–6 minutes, but the latency of tumour formation is long, ranging from 190 ± 80 days for cranial nerve tumours to 245 ± 80 days for cerebral gliomas [1]. Although much was known of the histology of such tumours, until recently little was known of the underlying mechanism of carcinogenesis beyond the fact that ENU was capable of alkylating DNA and was likely to be inducing genetic mutations.

In 1981, R.A. Weinberg and his colleagues subjected DNA prepared from a cell line called B104, derived from an ENU-induced rat neuroblastoma [2], to transfection onto mouse NIH-3T3 fibroblast cells [3]. Many foci of transformed cells were observed which were selected and grown out in culture. Of the 13 transfectant lines developed, all were tumourgenic in newborn mice. DNA prepared from these primary tranfectant lines were able to induce foci after a second cycle of transfection. Sera from animals bearing fibrosarcomas induced by injection of secondary transfectant cells precipitated a polypeptide of

185 000 molecular weight, called p185, present in the B104 cell line and all its transfection derived progeny [4]. This protein was not present in a variety of other transformed cell lines and it was thus hypothesised that p185 was encoded by the transforming sequence and that its expression might be responsible for transformation [4]. Subsequently it was found that four cell lines which had been independently derived by transfection of DNA from ENU-induced tumours had a common pattern of sensitivity to inactivation by restriction endonucleases and that each expressed the p185 protein, suggesting that the acquired gene was the same in each case. The name 'neu' was therefore applied to this gene, because of its common derivation from neuroblastomas.

DNA prepared from neu-containing cell lines was subjected to Southern blot analysis using a selection of, usually retrovirally encoded, oncogene probes to determine whether the neu gene was related to any of the previously identified sequences. An EcoRI fragment of DNA present in all the transfected cells but not in the parental NIH-3T3 fibroblasts was found to hybridise with, and therefore be structurally related to, the chicken v-erbB gene [5]. The v-erbB gene is a retrovirally transduced fragment of the chicken c-erbB1 gene which encodes the epidermal growth factor receptor protein. The EGF receptor is a transmembrane cell surface glycoprotein of 175 000 molecular weight which binds EGF, TGFα and related virally encoded growth factors. Ligand binding activates the intrinsic tyrosine kinase activity of the cytoplasmic domain of the EGF receptor leading to pleotropic effects on cells, including the stimulation of mitogenesis [6]. As discussed below, the neu gene thus appeared to encode a growth factor receptor-related molecule.

In order to determine by what mechanism the neu gene had become activated to an oncogene (onc-neu) it was necessary to compare its structure to its normal cellular counterpart, the c-neu proto-oncogene. To this end genomic clones encoding the transforming onc-neu gene and the c-neu gene were isolated. Restriction analysis indicated that both genes were encoded within 23–33 Kb fragments of DNA. The two cloned genes displayed identical restriction maps using several enzymes that cleaved at a total of 50 sites within the two sequences [7]. A cell line called DHFR-G8 containing 80–100 copies of the c-neu proto-oncogene was selected by co-transfection with the dihydrofolate reductase gene and subsequent growth in methotrexate. Despite this high level of c-neu gene amplification, which leads to a concomitant overexpression of the c-*neu* protein, the transfected cells were not morphologically altered.

Very recently, Di Fiore *et al.* have reported that expression of moderate levels of the normal human c-*erb*B2 protein, the human equivalent to the rat c-*neu* proto-oncogene, in immortalised but non-tumourigenic mouse NIH-3T3 cells were not transforming. However, higher levels of expression resulted in conversion of the cells to a very malignant phenotype [8]. Thus the level of expression of the c-*erb*B2 protein appears to be critical in determining whether the recipient cells become transformed. In contrast, however, even low levels of the *onc-neu* gene were fully transforming in the same cells, emphasising that the structurally subtle difference between the two rat genes was critical for transformation [7]. Subsequent work by Bargmann *et al.* demonstrated that a single point mutation was present in the *onc-neu* cDNA sequence leading to the conversion of a valine residue to a glutamic acid residue in the transmembrane domain of the c-*neu* protein and that this was the only difference between the molecules. The same point mutation was found in four independently derived lines containing activated *onc-neu*, confirming that this change alone was responsible for cell transformation, and indicating that this mutation may be a common consequence of ENU treatment [9, 10].

HUMAN C-*ERB*B2 AND ITS RELATIONSHIP TO C-*ERB*B1/EGFR

During the last two years the cDNA sequence of both rat c-*neu* [11] andits human counterpart, called either HER-2/*neu* [12] or c-*erb*B2 [13], have been determined. In both cases the homologous chicken retroviral v-*erb*B gene was used as a probe to isolate cDNA clones. Transcription of the normal rat c-*neu* gene gives a 4.4 Kb mRNA and the human c-*erb*B2 gene 4.6 Kb mRNA. The rat mRNA contains an open reading frame of 3780 nucleotides specifying a protein of 1280 amino acids, molecular weight 139 221. The human transcript encodes a protein of 1255 amino acids, molecular weight 137 895. Post-translational modification by glycosylation and phosphorylation of the rat and human c-*erb*B2 proteins results in their mature forms possessing molecular weights of 185 000 and 190 000 respectively. The predicted amino acid sequence of the two molecules is highly homologous (88% identity), the least homologous region being the putative transmembrane domain (55%).

The sequence of the human c-erbB2 gene product is highly homologous to the sequence of the human epidermal growth factor receptor (Fig. 3.1) [6, 10]. The EGF receptor is known to be a transmembrane protein with 621 amino acids being extracellular and 543 amino acids intracellular. At least some of the c-*neu* protein is expressed on the cell surface and so can be hypothesised also to be a membrane spanning molecule [14]. The sequences of the two molecules can be considered as co-linear. Comparison of the two reveals that their extracellular sequences are 43% homologous. This figure is perhaps misleading, however, since the 51 cysteine residues arranged in two repeating motifs in the EGF receptor are absolutely conserved in the c-erbB2 protein. Most of these residues are probably involved in forming disulphide bonds important to the assembly and stability of the molecules, strongly indicating a tertiary structural relationship in addition to a sequential one. Antibodies raised to denatured EGF receptors cross-react with the c-erbB2 protein emphasising their structural similarity [5].

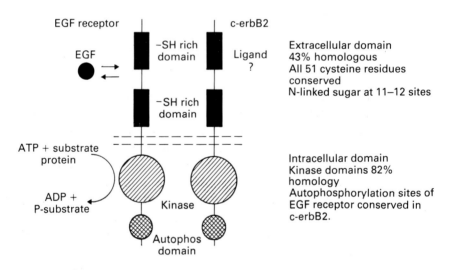

Fig. 3.1   Diagrammatic representation of the structure of the human EGF receptor and the c-erbB2 protein.

As with the limited homology between the transmembrane domains of rat c-*neu* and c-erbB2, the same lack of homology is apparent when comparing these regions with that of the EGF receptor where there is 27% homology between human EGF receptor and c-*erb*B2. The cytoplasmic sequences of the two molecules are, however, much more highly conserved, although regionally. Both molecules possess tyrosine kinase domains extending from 50 amino acids from the inner face of the membrane to about position 980 in the sequence. These regions are highly homologous with 82% of the amino acid sequence absolutely conserved. Downstream of the kinase domain and before the phosphorylation site domain, there are about 40 additional amino acids in the c-*erb*B2 protein which bear no structural relationship to any sequences in the EGF receptor. It will be interesting to see from the intron-exon boundaries in the gene whether these residues reside in a discrete exon or exons.

The c-*erb*B2 protein possesses three tyrosine residues near its carboxy terminus (C-terminus) in equivalent positions to the three which are known to be the major sites of autophosphorylation in the EGF receptor. Although both *neu* [15] and c-*erb*B2 [16] have been shown to possess tyrosine kinase activity by their ability to autophosphorylate in an immune complex assay, it is not presently known whether these residues are sites of modification.

AMPLIFICATION OF THE C-*ERB*B GENES IN HUMAN TUMOURS

The rat c-*neu* gene can be activated by a point mutation to a dominantly transforming oncogene. What of its human counterpart, the c-*erb*B2 gene? Despite many attempts, no transforming version of the c-*erb*B2 gene has been detected by DNA transfections from human tumours. This does not necessarily mean that such activating mutations do not occur. More likely, the transfection assay is incapable of detecting such altered genes should they exist because they are, as discussed in the introduction, too large to be transferred intact into the recipient cells. The human c-*erb*B1/EGFR gene is 110 kb in length, possessing 25 intron sequences, and the c-*erb*B2 gene may be equally large. Sequences of larger than 50–100 kb are transfected very inefficiently.

Parenthetically, it is a curious point that several genes encoding molecules related to growth factor receptors and apparently encoding protein tyrosine kinase activity such as *ret* [17] and *raf* [18] have been activated to oncogenes by recombination or fragmentation occurring during the transfection process. Examination of the original tumour DNA showed the presence of what appeared to be normal gene copies.

Activated versions of the c-*erb*B1/EGFR and c-*erb*B2 genes have never been detected in this way although N-terminal truncation of the EGF receptor is known to be sufficient to activate it to an oncogene under certain circumstances and truncation of c-*erb*B2 enhances its trans-forming potential [8]. Recent evidence suggests however that both N-terminal and C-terminal truncation of the EGF receptor are required for it to transform a wider range of normal recipient cell types. Why such truncated, transforming versions of these genes have not so far been produced artificially by transfection is intriguing.

What has been observed with both the c-*erb*B1/EGFR and c-*erb*B2 genes is that they are frequently amplified in human tumours such that a single tumour cell may possess as many as 20 or more times the gene copy number found in normal cells. This chapter will concen-trate on the c-*erb*B2 gene and those tumours in which amplification and/or overexpression of the protein has occurred. However, a com-parison of these events to the situation in which the c-*erb*B1/EGFR gene is amplified or overexpressed may be additionally instructive. Technically, the analysis of gene amplification *per se* is simple, how-ever, gene rearrangements that may occur during amplification are a more complex phenomenon to dissect. Evidence to date suggests that gene rearrangement associated with gene amplification does occur within the c-*erb*B1/EGFR and c-*erb*B2 sequences in human tumours, but at a rather low frequency compared with amplification alone and it may be more common among, or confined to, certain tumour types. Because only one such event has been analysed in any detail, re-arrangements will not be discussed in depth here. Amplification of the c-*erb*B2 gene has been found in breast [19–24], stomach [25], kidney [21] and salivary gland adenocarcinomas [26] (Table 3.1). Breast

Table 3.1   Occurrence of c-*erb*B2 gene amplification in various human tumours

Tumour type	Occurence	Reference
Breast adenocarcinomas	94/371	19–24
Stomach adenocarcinomas	3/10	25
Salivary adenocarcinomas	1/1	26
Kidney adenocarcinomas	1/4	21
Colon adenocarcinomas	1/96	21, 27*
Squamous cell carcinomas	0/8	21
Sarcomas	0/9	21
Leukaemias	0/21	21

*P. Johnson, D.J. Venter, W.J. Gullick and D.N. Carney (unpublished results)

Table 3.2 Summary of c-*erb*B2 gene amplification in human breast adenocarcinomas

Fold amplification		
2–5	> 5	Reference
53/189 (28%)	27/189 (14%)	19
16/95 (17%)	0/95 (0%)	23
12/36 (33%)	6/36 (17%)	22
13/51 (25%)	3/51 (6%)	24
Total: 94/371 (25%)	36/371 (10%)	

adenocarcinomas have been the main focus of attention so far, partly because they are a common human tumour, frequently removed surgically, and thus available for analysis, and partly because of the observed high frequency of amplification. In the largest group studied to date, Slamon *et al*. 53 of 189 (28%) of tumours contained amplified c-*erb*B2 genes [19], a figure now bracketed by other studies (12 of 36 (33%) [22]; 16 of 95 (17%) [23]; 13 of 51 (25%) [24]) (Table 3.2). Generally one restriction endonuclease has been used in these studies and thus only gross gene re-arrangements would be detected; however, Slamon *et al*. suggested that two of the 53 tumours with amplification had been subject to re-arrangement. The extent of amplification varied but for correlative analysis with other parameters Slamon *et al*. divided tumours with amplification into three categories, 2–5, 6–20, and > 20-fold amplification. Taking all the studies together and using these arbitrary divisions, roughly 10% of the total tumours contained 2–5 copies, 10% 6–20, and 5% > 20 copies (Table 3.2). Only four of the 189 tumours examined by Slamon *et al*. contained amplified copies of the c-*erb*B1/EGFR gene. Since nearly 400 breast tumours have now been examined at the DNA level, these figures are likely to remain relatively unchanged.

It is not presently possible to assess the frequency of c-*erb*B2 gene amplification in other tumour types since so far inadequate numbers have been examined. One exception to this, however, is in the area of colonic adenocarcinomas where three series of tumours have been examined, 29 by Yokota *et al*. 1986 [21], 22 by P. Johnson, D.J. Venter, D.N. Carney and W.J. Gullick (unpublished results), and 45 by Meltzer *et al*. [27]. Only one of these 96 tumours examined showed amplification of the c-*erb*B2 gene. Yokota *et al*. have also demonstrated that amplification occurs infrequently, or not at all, in squamous cell tumours, sarcomas and leukaemias (Table 3.2). Tumours derived from transitional epithelium such as bladder have yet to be examined. These results give a preliminary indication that amplification of this gene may be confined to certain tumour types.

In contrast, the c-*erb*B1/EGFR gene has been found to be amplified mostly in squamous cell carcinomas and brain tumours, and occasionally in adenocarcinomas. Only one of 32 (3%) bladder tumours [28], two of ten (20%) squamous tumours of the lung [29] and four of ten (40%) glioblastoma multiformae [30] contained amplified c-*erb*B1/EGFR genes. In the case of both the c-*erb*B1/EGFR and c-*erb*B2 genes, these figures of amplification frequencies are generally derived from relatively small numbers of specimens. More numerically extensive and wider ranging analyses should provide a more general picture, which ultimately should be of interest to epidemiologists.

In addition to changes in the c-*erb*B genes themselves, other genetic changes inevitably occur during gene amplification. Van de Vijver *et al*. [23] have reported that the human c-*erb*A gene, the cognate in humans of the chicken v-*erb*A gene, was co-amplified in six of ten tumours with amplified c-*erb*B2 genes. This result might have represented a situation of co-operative behaviour of two protooncogene products, in this case probably as a consequence of serendipitous co-amplification which is due to genetic linkage as the two genes map to the same band on human chromosome 17, q21. However, the possibility of co-operation appears unlikely in this case because the authors also report that despite high levels of c-*erb*B2 mRNA there was no detectable expression of the c-*erb*A gene. This finding does, however, emphasise that the amplicon size in human gene amplification events can be very large, in extreme cases as much as 10^7 base pairs [31, 32], representing 5% of an average sized chromosome. Thus, if the c-*erb*B2 gene is approximately 100 kb, it would represent only 1% of an amplified unit of this size. Other co-amplified genes may not necessarily co-operate in transformation but on the other hand their overexpression must not be lethal. Does this condition impose constraints on amplification of some proto-oncogenes in different differentiated cell types? Perhaps in cells where c-*erb*A is normally expressed, amplification might affect the cells' phenotype, whereas if the gene is normally transcriptionally silent amplification is likely to be inconsequential. The chromosomal location of particular proto-oncogenes differs between species and thus consideration of possible co-amplification of neighbouring genes will be species-dependent. In addition, since presumably the selective pressure for c-*erb*B2 gene amplification is (in contrast to the results of drug resistance studies) a positive selection for overgrowth of particular clones of tumour cells, why are some tissues apparently more prone to this than others? Are breast epithelial cells for instance more capable of responding to over-expression of the c-*erb*B2 protein than other differentiated cell types?

As discussed below, some tissues display amplification of the c-*erb*B1/EGFR gene, whereas others overexpress the protein without evidence of gross genetic change, probably mediated instead by alterations in transcriptional control. The c-*erb*B2 gene on the other hand seems to be overexpressed principally, if not exclusively, in association with gene amplification. Studies on drug resistance may throw light on this difference in behaviour. Drug resistance is usually a consequence of gene amplification but one exception to this is resistance to canavanine [32, 33] in fibroblasts where cells were selected that had increased their rate of transcription of the normal gene leading to increased protein synthesis. This gene, encoding the enzyme argininosuccinate synthetase, is normally expressed at high levels only in liver cells. It may be that where a mechanism exists for a wide variation in the level of gene expression, such a mechanism may be activated, perhaps by mutation. Where a gene has little ability to have its rate of mRNA synthesis controlled the only available way that increased levels of protein can be achieved is by amplification, thereby increasing the number of transcribing units. The EGF receptor can be synthesised at widely varying levels in different tissues whereas some evidence has suggested that c-*erb*B2 protein expression may be more constant [36]. The promoter sequences of the EGF receptor and c-*erb*B2 genes are completely different in structure [34, 35]. Therefore, it is possible that these differences in the control mechanisms for transcription influence the frequency of appearance of particular types of abnormal activated events, such as gene amplification versus deregulation of transcription.

Finally, the question arises as to how uniform gene amplification is amongst a given group of tumour cells. Several alternatives are possible. Firstly there may exist a level of gene amplification which is homogenous throughout a particular tumour but this level differs in extent between tumours. Secondly, there may be a homogeneous level of amplification only in some cells within a tumour and that this proportion varies between tumours. Finally, it could be that different levels of gene amplification are present in individual cells in any tumour.

These alternatives are important for mechanistic reasons. For instance, are there multiple rounds of gene amplification or a single episode? Are low levels of gene amplification as measured by Southern blotting sometimes misleading in that they do not detect small populations of tumour cells which contain extensively amplified genes, and is this prognostically significant? Amplified genes are frequently present at chromosomal locations which are different from where the normal gene resides. The position in the genome may influence the extent of transcription but this variation could not be recognised by Southern blotting alone. Several of these questions can be answered by examining the level and cellular pattern of expression of the protein encoded by the amplified gene, as it is the protein which is ultimately biologically active.

EXPRESSION OF THE C-*ERB*B1 AND 2 PROTEINS IN HUMAN TUMOURS

As discussed in the previous section, there are observable differences in frequency of amplification of the c-*erb*B2 gene between different tumour types. In addition, the c-*erb*B1/EGFR gene, although amplified in certain types of tumours, is more frequently activated by some other mechanism to produce overexpression of the protein it encodes. Thus, two questions arise concerning the c-*erb*B2 system. Firstly, is the c-*erb*B2 protein overexpressed in the tumour cells of biopsies of human tumours which contain amplified c-*erb*B2 genes? Secondly, are there examples of overexpression of the c-*erb*B2 protein in tumours in the absence of gene amplification?

In order to address these questions, it was necessary to develop antibodies that recognise the human c-*erb*B2 protein by immunohistological staining of thin sections of human tumour biopsies. Venter *et al.* [22] recently reported the use of such reagents to stain a series of human breast adenocarcinomas and the level of staining intensity was compared with the c-*erb*B2 gene status. Twelve of 36 (33%) of the tumours contained detectable c-*erb*B2 gene amplification. Using an antibody raised to a synthetic peptide derived from the predicted c-*erb*B2 protein sequence, it was shown that in this series of tumours those with gene amplification stained prominently but those without amplification gave lower or negligible staining. A very weak or negligible reaction was seen on normal breast tissue (Fig. 3.2). These results were confirmed by Western blot analysis [22]. A subsequent

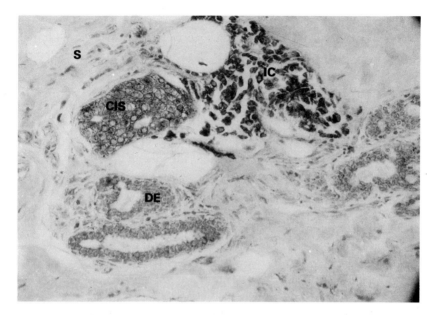

Fig. 3.2   Staining of a thin section of a paraffin embedded human breast carcinoma with an antibody raised to a synthetic peptide from the sequence of the c-*erb*B2 protein. There is very slight staining of the normal ductal epithelium (DE) and stroma (S). The area of invasive carcinoma (IC) shows strong staining, while the area of carcinoma *in situ* (CIS) shows an intermediate staining intensity.

study by van de Vijver *et al.* (R. Nusse, personal communication), using a similar antibody to stain a series of breast adenocarcinomas, gave essentially concordant results. Other work by Berger *et al.* [24] showed strong staining of breast tumours with gene amplification but also some staining on tumours without amplification.

The only other type of tumours which have been stained for expression of the c-*erb*B2 protein at the time of writing are a series of colonic adenocarcinomas without evidence of gene amplification (P. Johnson, D.J. Venter, D.N. Carney and W.J. Gullick, unpublished results). The staining pattern obtained was variable between individual tumours, but generally moderate or low in intensity.

Thus the answer to the first question posed earlier is that essentially all tumours with moderate to high levels of gene amplification give strong staining reactions. Interestingly, the subcellular pattern of staining showed, in addition to the expected cell surface expression, a degree of intracellular staining that was punctate in appearance.

This probably represents the c-*erb*B2 protein since two antibodies raised to different sequences from the c-*erb*B2 protein give similar intracellular staining patterns (B. Gusterson and W.J. Gullick, unpublished results). The role of this apparently intracellular c-*erb*B2 protein is not known.

As for expression of the c-*erb*B2 protein in tumours without detectable gene amplification, the data to date suggest that this may possibly occur but it is generally at a lower level than that associated with gene amplification. A study by Kraus *et al.* showed that of 13 breast cell lines examined, five expressed equivalently low levels of c-*erb*B2 mRNA, four had four to eight-fold higher levels and four contained 64–128 fold levels [37]. The latter four lines showed c-*erb*2 gene amplification, whereas all the others contained apparently normal numbers of c-*erb*B2 genes. Thus, these authors suggest that two mechanisms can lead to elevated expression of the c-*erb*B2 protein, one involving increased transcription, leading to moderately elevated protein expression, and one in which gene amplification results in very high levels of protein expression. The same situation may occur in human malignancies. It is, however, difficult to prove that the presence of a four to eight-fold higher level of c-*erb*B2 mRNA in one cell type versus another is actually an aberrant, abnormal event. It might alternatively represent a normal phenomenon associated with the differentiated phenotype of the cell. The availability of antibodies that can detect the c-*erb*B2 protein in tissues embedded in paraffin wax should allow many more common and uncommon tumours to be examined. It also provides a method of testing the hypothesis proposed by Slamon *et al.* that the presence of abnormal levels of c-*erb*B2 in breast cancers indicate a short time disease free interval and poor survival [19].

The c-*erb*B2 gene is amplified in other types of tumours, including kidney [21], salivary gland [26], stomach [25] (Table 3.1), and in lung adenocarcinomas (M. Cline, personal communication). As yet no analysis of the level of expression of the c-*erb*B2 protein in these types of cancers has been reported, however, such studies may be anticipated. These analyses are preliminary and over the next few years much more information will emerge allowing more accurate generalisations as to the frequency and extent of aberrant c-*erb*B2 expression in various tumour types. Whether this will provide a clinically useful marker for predicting tumour progression remains to be determined but since overexpression of the normal c-*erb*B2 protein is capable of transforming non-malignant, but immortalised cells in culture [8], it may well play a role in causing or sustaining the transformed state of some human tumours.

CONCLUSIONS

The discovery in a chemically induced rat neuroblastoma of the *neu* oncogene has allowed the analysis of its human counterpart, the c-*erbB*2 gene, in normal and transformed human cells and primary tumour biopsies. The gene, which encodes a molecule closely related to the human EGF receptor, is frequently amplified in certain types of human adenocarcinomas, leading to the overexpression of the c-*erbB*2 protein. Experiments using cultured cells have shown that artificial overexpression of the normal human c-*erbB*2 protein is sufficient to transform cells. Studies are underway to elucidate the role of the c-*erbB*2 protein in human tumours. Some indications exist that the presence of elevated levels of c-*erbB*2 protein in human breast cancer may be an indicator of prognosis. Overexpression of this cell surface molecule opens up the possibility of exploiting this phenomenon to specifically localise human tumours by imaging techniques. In the light of the demonstration that treatment of cells expressing the mutated, transforming, *neu* protein with a monoclonal antibody, either in culture [38] or as established tumours in animals [39] leads to cytotoxicity and inhibition of tumour growth, similar approaches may prove fruitful in attempts to treat tumours in humans.

REFERENCES

1 Lantos, P.L. Development of nitrosourea-induced brain tumours—with a special note on changes occurring during latency. *Fd Chem Toxic.* 1986, **24**: 121–127.

2 Schubert, D., Heinemann, S., Carlisle, W. *et al.* Clonal cell lines from the rat central nervous system. *Nature.* 1974, **249**: 224–227.

3 Shih, C., Padhy, L.C., Murray, M. and Weinberg, R.A. Transforming genes of carcinomas and neuroblastomas introduced into mouse fibroblasts. *Nature.* 1981, **20**: 261–264.

4 Padhy, L.C., Shih, C., Cowing, D., Finkelstein, R. and Weinberg, R.A. Identification of a phosphoprotein specifically induced by the transforming DNA of a rat neuroblastomas. *Cell.* 1982, **28**: 865–871.

5 Schecter, A.L., Hung, M.C., Vaidyanathan, L. *et al.* The neu gene: an erbB-homologous gene distinct from and unlinked to the gene encoding the EGF receptor. *Science.* 1985, **229**: 976–978.

6 Gullick, W.J. and Waterfield, M.D. Epidermal growth factor and its receptor. In: Strasberg, A.D., (ed.) *Molecular Biology of Receptors.* Chichester: Ellis Horwood, 1987, 15–35.

7 Hung, M.C., Schechter, A.L., Chevray, P-Y. M., Stern, D.F. and Weinberg, R.A. Molecular cloning of the neu gene: Absence of gross structural alteration in oncogenic alleles. *Proc Natl Acad Sci USA*. 1986, **83**: 261–264.

8 Di Fiore, P.P., Pierce, J.H., Kraus, M.H., Segatto, O., King, C.R. and Aaronson, S.A. erbB-2 is a potent oncogene when overexpressed in NIH/3T3 cells. *Science*. 1987, **237**: 178–182.

9 Bargmann, C.I., Hung, M.C. and Weinberg, R.A. Multiple independent activation of the neu oncogenes by a point mutation altering the transmembrane domain of p185. *Cell*. 1986, **45**: 649–657.

10 Gullick, W.J. A comparison of the structures of single polypeptide chain growth factor receptors that possess protein tyrosine kinase activity. In: Cooke, B.A., King, R.J.V., and van der Molen (eds) *Hormones and their Actions*. Amsterdam: Elsevier, 1988, 349–360.

11 Bergmann, C.I., Hung, M.C. and Weinberg, R.A. The neu oncogene encodes an epidermal growth factor receptor-related protein. *Nature*. 1986, **319**: 230–234.

12 Coussens, L., Yang-Feng, T.L., Liao, Y-C *et al*. Tyrosine kinase receptor with extensive homology to EGF receptor shares chromosomal location with neu oncogene. *Science*. 1985, **230**: 1132–1139.

13 Yamamoto, T., Ikawa, S., Akiyama, T., *et al*. Similarity of protein encoded by the human c-erbB-2 gene to epidermal growth factor receptor. *Nature*. 1986, **319**: 226–230.

14 Drebin, J.A., Stern, D.F., Link, V.C., Weinberg, R.A. and Greene, M.I. Monoclonal antibodies identify a cell-surface antigen associated with an activated cellular oncogene. *Nature*. 1984, **312**: 545–548.

15 Stern, D.F., Heffernan, P.A. and Weinberg, R.A. p185, a product of the neu proto-oncogene, is a receptor-like protein associated with tyrosine kinase activity. *Mol Cell Biol*. 1986, **6**: 1729–1740.

16 Akiyama, T., Sudo, C., Ogawara, H., Toyoshima, K. and Yamamoto, T. The product of the human c-erbB-2 gene: a 185-kilodalton glycoprotein with tyrosine kinase activity. *Science*. 1986, **232**: 1644–1646.

17 Takahashi, M. and Cooper, G.M. Ret transforming gene encodes a fusion protein homologous to tyrosine kinases. *Mol Cell Biol*. 1987, **7**: 1378–1385.

18 Stanton, V.P. and Cooper, G.M. Activation of human raf transforming genes by deletion of normal amino-terminal coding sequences. *Mol Cell Biol*. 1987, **7**: 1171–1179.

19 Slamon, D.J., Clark, G.M., Wong, S.G., Levin, W.J., Ullrich, A. and McGuire, W.L. Human breast cancer: correlation of relapse and survival with amplification of the HER-2/neu oncogene. *Science*. 1987, **235**: 177–182.

20 King, C.R., Kraus, M.H. and Aaronson, S.A. Amplification of a novel v-erbB-related gene in a human mammary carcinoma. *Science*. 1985, **229**: 974–976.

21 Yokota, J., Yamamoto, T., Toyoshima, K, *et al*. Amplification of c-erbB-2 oncogene in human adenocarcinomas *in vivo*. *Lancet* 1986, **i**: 765–766.

22 Venter, D.J., Tuzi, N.L., Kumar, S. and Gullick, W.J. Overexpression of the c-erbB-2 oncoprotein in human breast carcinomas: Immunohistological assessment correlates with gene amplification. *Lancet*. 1987, **ii**: 69–72.

23 Van de Vijver, M., Van de Bersselaar, R., Devilee, P., Cornelisse, C., Peterse, J. and Nusse, R. Amplification of the neu (c-erbB-2) oncogene in human mammary tumours is relatively frequent and is often accompanied by amplification of the linked c-erbA oncogene. *Mol Cell Biol*. 1987, **7**: 2019–2023.

24 Berger, M.S., Locher, G.W., Saurer, S., Gullick, W.J., Waterfield, M.D., Groner, B. and Hynes, N.E. C-erbB-2 gene amplification and protein expression in human breast carcinoma correlates with nodal status and nuclear grading. *Cancer Res.* 1988, **48**: 1238–1242.

25 Fukushige, S-I., Matsubara, K-I., Yoshida, M., *et al.* Localisation of a novel v-erbB-related gene, c-erbB-2, on human chromosome 17 and its amplification in a gastric cancer cell line. *Mol Cell Biol.* 1986, **6**: 955–958.

26 Semba, K., Kamata, N., Toyoshima, K. and Yamamoto, T. A v-erbB related proto-oncogene, c-erbB-2, is distinct from the c-erbB-1/epidermal growth factor-receptor gene and is amplified in a human salivary gland adenocarcinoma. *Proc Natl Acad Sci USA.* 1985, **82**: 6497–6501.

27 Meltzer, S.J., Ahnen, D.J., Battifora, H., Yokota, J. and Cline, M.J. Proto-oncogene abnormalities in colon cancers and adenomatous polyps. *Gastroenterology.* 1987, **92**: 1174–1180.

28 Berger, M.S., Greenfield, C., Gullick, W.J. *et al.* Evaluation of epidermal growth factor receptors in bladder tumours. *Br J Can.* 1987, **56**: 533–537.

29 Berger, M.S., Gullick, W.J., Greenfield, C., Evans, S., Addis, B.J. and Waterfield, M.D. Epidermal growth factor receptors in lung tumours. *J Pathol.* 1987, **152**: 297–307.

30 Libermann, T.A., Nusbaum, H.R., Razon, N., *et al.* Amplification, enhanced expression and possible rearrangement of EGF receptor gene in primary human brain tumours of glial origin. *Nature.* 1985, **313**: 144–147.

31 Stark, G.R. and Wahl, G.M. Gene amplification. *Annu Rev Biochem.* 1984, **53**: 447–491.

32 Stark, G.R. DNA amplification in drug resistant cells and in tumours. *Cancer Surv.* 1986, **5**: 1–23.

33 Su, T.S., Bock, H-G. O., O'Brien, W.E. and Beaudet, A.L. Cloning of cDNA for argininosuccinate synthetase mRNA and study of enzyme overproduction in a human cell line. *J Biol Chem.* 1981, **256**: 11826–11831.

34 Tal, M., King, C.R., Kraus, M.H., Ullrich, A., Schlessinger, J. and Givol, D. Human HER2 (neu) promoter: Evidence for multiple mechanisms for transcriptional initiation. *Mol Cell Biol.* 1987, **7**: 2597–2601.

35 Ishii, S., Inamoto, F., Yamanashi, Y., Togoshima, K. and Yamamoto, T. Characterisation of the promoter region of the human c-erbB-2 oncogene. *Proc Natl Acad Sci USA.* 1987, **84**: 4374–4378.

36 Gullick, W.J., Berger, M.S., Bennett, P.L.P., Rothbard, J.B. and Waterfield, M.D. Expression of the c-erbB-2 protein in normal and transformed cells. *Int J Can.* 1987, **40**: 246–254.

37 Kraus, M.H., Popescu, N.C., Amsbaugh, S.C. and King, C.R. Overexpression of the EGF receptor-relaated proto-oncogene erbB-2 in human mammary tumour cell lines by different molecular mechanisms. *EMBO J.* 1987, **6**: 605–610.

38 Drebin, J.A., Link, V.C., Stern, D.F., Weinberg, R.A. and Greene, M.I. Down-modulation of an oncogene protein product and reversion of the transformed phenotype by monoclonal antibodies. *Cell.* 1985, **41**: 695–706.

39 Drebin, J.A., Link, V.C., Weinberg, R.A. and Greene, M.I. Inhibition of tumour growth by a monoclonal antibody reactive with an oncogene-encoded tumour antigen. *Proc Natl Acad Sci USA.* 1986, **83**: 9129–9133.

4 BOMBESIN AND ITS RECEPTOR

D.N. CARNEY

Bⁿᵒᵐᵇᵉˢⁱⁿ (BN) a 14 amino acid peptide was first isolated from the skin of the European frog *Bombina bombina* in 1972. Subsequently it was found that structurally related peptides such as alytensin (14 amino acids) litorin (nine amino acids) and ranatensin (11 amino acids) were present in extracts of skin from other amphibian species. More recently, in 1979 a 27 amino acid peptide, gastrin releasing peptide (GRP) was isolated from porcine stomach tissue and purified.

GRP has been shown to have the same COOH-terminal decapeptide as bombesin with the exception of a single amino acid substitution [1–3] (Fig. 4.1). When injected into laboratory animals GRP produces the same constellation of effects as bombesin. For these reasons GRP is considered to be the mammalian homologue of amphibian bombesin [3]. Data also suggests that bombesin and GRP interact with the same cellular receptors, and the homologous carboxy-terminal region in both peptides is responsible for receptor recognition. In addition the similarity between bombesin and GRP results in common antigens shared by both which can be demonstrated by polyclonal antisera.

Using a variety of antibodies to BN/GRP, bombesin-like immunoreactivity (BLI) has been demonstrated in mammalian gastrointestinal tract tissues, brain, spinal cord and lung. Immunohistochemical studies have shown BLI to be present in nerve fibres of the mammalian gastrointestinal tract, and in the endocrine cells of both avian and amphibian stomach. A corresponding peptide to GRP has also been isolated from chicken stomach, differing from the porcine GRP in nine of 27 residues, but with an identical carboxy-terminal octapeptide sequence [4]. BLI like peptides have been found in several forms in the canine gastrointestinal tract. One of these peptides contains a 27 amino acid residue which is homologous in structure to porcine GRP with minor differences at positions 4, 5, 7 and 12, but not in the biologically active carboxy-terminal monopeptide of the protein.

BLI is also present in human foetal lung and is located in pulmonary endocrine cells [5, 6]. The concentrations of these peptides is higher

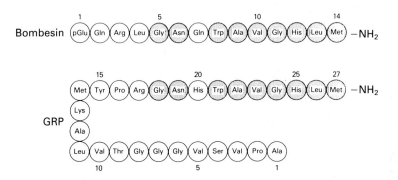

Fig. 4.1   Amino acid sequence of bombesin and GRP.

in foetal than neonatal lung, suggesting a role for these peptides in lung development. This immunoreactivity for BLI is detectable in foetal lung at the twelfth gestational week and is related to the carboxy-terminal fraction of GRP rather than the whole 27 amino acids of GRP or bombesin [5]. In the human lung BLI co-localises with calcitonin-like immunoreactivity in both adult and foetal tissues [6].

Bombesin and GRP have been shown to display a variety of potent direct and indirect actions on gut secretions and motility and on the central nervous system. Intravenous infusions of bombesin produce a wide variety of actions in mammals including stimulation of pancreatic enzyme secretion, gallbladder contraction, antidiuresis, increase in systolic blood pressure, and increased gastrointestinal motility [2, 4]. Intracisternal administration in rats causes hypothermia and hyperglycaemia. In addition infusion of bombesin results in increased prolactin and growth hormone secretion from the pituitary gland in the pig, rat and human pituitary.

Thus investigation of a range of tissues in different animal species have demonstrated BN/GRP like peptides to be widely distributed. Their conservation in evolution coupled with their widespread distribution suggests they have important physiological and pharmacological roles. As their actions appear to be mediated by binding to specific high affinity binding receptors, a better understanding of the exact role of these peptides in normal healthy states may be of potential therapeutic value in those situations where there is disordered regulation of these peptides and/or their receptors.

CHROMOSOME LOCALISATION OF GRP GENE

Several studies have recently reported on the localisation of the GRP gene [7–10]. Genomic blotting has shown that the human GRP cDNA' probe hybridised to three HindIII fragments (11.0 kb, 4.6 kb and 2.9 kb) and to three BamHI fragments (14.5 kb, 11.0 kb and 2.7 kb) in human genomic DNA. Southern blotting experiments using mouse and hamster DNA have revealed species specific fragments homologous to the GRP probe. This species difference has led to work on somatic cell hybrids which has attempted to localise the gene for GRP. Using restriction fragment mapping to genomic DNA from somatic cell hybrids Naylor et al. [7] localised the human gene of GRP to chromosome 18. Using a panel of rodent-human somatic cell hybrid cell lines the localisation of the gene to chromosome 18 has been confirmed [8]. Moreover, in situ chromosomal hybridisation studies further mapped the GRP gene to chromosome band 18q21.

BN/GRP are growth factors for small cell lung cancer (SCLC). Cytogenetic abnormalities of genes encoding oncogenes, growth factor receptors or growth factors have been demonstrated in many different human tumours. In SCLC cells the most consistent and, indeed, specific chromosome abnormality is a deletion of the short arm of chromosome 3. While changes involving other chromosomes have occasionally been noted, they are not specific nor consistent. Thus far, abnormalities of chromosome 18, the site of the GRP gene, have not been identified in SCLC, suggesting that in this tumour, chromosomal abnormalities do not affect the GRP structural gene. Moreover, re-arrangement or amplification of the GRP structural gene in SCLC tumours have not been observed.

Cloning of mRNA from tumours has established that human GRP is encoded in a polypeptide precursor that contains a single copy of GRP. Using RNA from a pulmonary carcinoid Spindel et al. [11] obtained DNA clones for the pre-pro GRP gene. Analysis of these clones revealed a pre-pro-GRP translation product consisting of a signal sequence (amino acids -23 to -1 GRP (amino acids 1–27) and a GRP-associated peptide (amino acids 31–125) of unknown function. Two types of pre-pro-GRP cDNA clones were observed in pulmonary carcinoid tissue which differed in the presence of a 19-base insertion in the 3' GRP-associated peptide occurring after amino acid 98 in pro-GRP. This alteration would provide for at least two forms of pro-GRP, differing in the carboxy-terminal GRP-associated peptide.

Following this investigation of the GRP gene in pulmonary carcinoids further analyses of this gene were carried out in SCLC cells
[9]. In SCLC a marked correlation was noted between pre-pro-GRP
gene expression and the occurrence of BLI in human SCLC cells.
These experiments also showed that SCLC cells *in vitro* produce at
least three different potential pre-pro-GRP RNAs as opposed to the
two types noted in carcinoids [9]. These structural differences appeared to arise after processing. The structure of the cDNAs of these
transcripts suggested alternative splicing, involving at least two donor
and acceptor sites. Nine SCLC cell lines were evaluated. Five contained
BLI and had evidence of pre-pro-GRP gene expression. Negative cell
lines had either c-*myc* or N-*myc* amplification and lacked neuroendocrine features. Thus, in SCLC, pre-pro-GRP gene expression may
serve as a marker of neuroendocrine differentiation.

The role of these different GRP associated peptides derived from
cDNA clones in SCLC is unclear. It is possible that the different forms
may have individual or specific physiological effects, or affect the
processing of the GRP prohormones. Further work is required to
establish their exact significance in SCLC cells.

Using highly specific antipeptide antisera raised against the synthetic peptides generated from regions along the predicted amino acid
sequence of pre-pro-GRP, the presence of GRP gene associated peptides (GGAPs) was evaluated in SCLC cell lines [10, 12]. Immunological assessment of SCLC whole cell lysates demonstrated GRP activity
at a molecular weight of 14–18 000, and GGAPs activity at molecular
weights of 14 000 and 8 000 and 27–28 000. These GGAPs were absent
in non-SCLC lung cancers and malignant melanoma lines. It has been
shown that the majority of primary SCLC tumours expressed GRP
and GGAPs. While there is no known biological function associated
with these GGAPs, their presence may serve as a marker for SCLC,
and it may be that they have as yet an undescribed biological role in
SCLC tumours.

Human GRP gene expression has been assessed in SCLC using a
cRNA probe. In both biopsy specimens fixed in paraformaldehyde,
and SCLC cell lines, hybridisation of pro-GRP was detected in tumour
cells in all specimens, providing evidence for the expression of the
pro-GRP gene in SCLC cells at a cellular level and showing that pro-
GRP gene mRNA is highly expressed in these tumours [13]. These *in
situ* hybridisation studies provide a means for evaluating pro-GRP
mRNA activity and functional morphology in fresh specimens of SCLC.

MECHANISM OF ACTION OF BOMBESIN/GASTRIN RELEASING PEPTIDE (BN/GRP)

Bombesin like peptides play an important role in regulating cellular proliferation in both normal and malignant cells. Their role as putative 'autocrine' growth factors in SCLC stresses the importance of understanding how these peptides regulate cell proliferation. It has long been recognized that cell surface receptors detect external signals and generate second messengers, such as C'AMP which control intracellular processes. An imbalance of second messengers may lead to abnormal cell behaviour and malignant change. In recent years, progress has been made in understanding the mechanism of action of an alternate system of message transduction involving receptors that generate intracellular signals from inositol lipids. One of these lipids, phosphatidylinositol 4,5 biphosphate is hydrolysed to diacylglycerol and inositol triphosphate as part of a signal transduction mechanism controlling a variety of cellular processes. Diacylglycerol acts within the membrane to activate protein kinase C, whereas inositol triphosphate leads to calcium flux [14].

The effects of bombesin on mammalian cells has been linked to changes in inositol phosphate production and calcium metabolism [15–17]. In Swiss 3T3 cells Takuwa et al. [15] evaluated the effect of bombesin on calcium metabolism and the turnover of phosphoinositides. Bombesin stimulates the breakdown of phosphatidylinositol 4,5 biphosphate, the production of inositol triphosphates and diaglycerol, and causes a transient elevation of intracellular free calcium. These studies clearly demonstrated that bombesin acts as a typical calcium messenger system hormone. It has also been postulated that the receptor stimulation of inositol phospholipid metabolism is mediated through a guanine nucleotide regulatory protein (Gp). Wakelam et al. [16] suggest that a plasma membrane protein p21, encoded by the N-ras proto-oncogene couples the receptors for growth factors including bombesin to the stimulation of phospholipases. Thus, expression of the p21 may stimulate cell growth by altering the sensitivity of cells to exogenous growth factors. An increase in coupling of these agents to phospholipases indicates how mutants of this oncogene may affect cellular proliferation in the malignant state.

Addition of bombesin to SCLC cells grown in culture increased cytoplasmic free calcium within seconds [17]. The increased calcium was derived in part from internal stores as the calcium shift could only be partially inhibited by EDTA. GRP (1–27) and GRP (20–27) were active in eliciting the response while GRP (1–16) and desleu[13]-met[14] bombesin (a weakly binding analogue of bombesin) were inactive. Coupled to the mobilisation of calcium, generation of inositol (1,4,5) triphosphate with delayed appearance of inositol (1,3,4) triphosphate occurred subsequent to bombesin treatment. Of interest, three of 79 responding SCLC cell lines were L-myc^+, c-myc^- and N-myc^- and expressed pre-pro-GRP mRNA. Six non-responding SCLC lines were all amplified for either c-myc or N-myc and expressed little or no pre-pro-GRP mRNA. Thus these data not only confirm that BN/GRP acts in a similar manner in SCLC cells as in 3T3 cells, but that activity in these cells may be linked to the amplification of genes of the myc family in that c-myc or N-myc over-expression appears to be associated with loss of GRP production and responsiveness in SCLC cell lines [17].

BOMBESIN/GRP: POTENT MITOGENS FOR CELLULAR PROLIFERATION

Much data exists which indicates that BN/GRP, in addition to exerting the wide range of physiological effects outlined above, are potent mitogens for a variety of cell types [18–23]. *In vivo* studies have shown that repeated administration of bombesin, induced pancreatic hyperplasia in rats, suggesting that bombesin could be an important peptide in the control or regulation of cell proliferation.

However, these *in vivo* observations could not clearly confirm that bombesin itself was responsible in that the hyperplasia observed could have resulted from the release of many other peptides as a consequence of bombesin administration. Thus, further studies have been carried out on a variety of *in vitro* models including Swiss 3T3 cells, rat pituitary cells and lung cancer cell lines.

Bombesin has been shown to stimulate the growth of Swiss 3T3 cells [18]. In these cells the effect was both disease and time dependent, with half-maximal effect observed at 1 nM. The effects of bombesin were observed both at a low serum concentration, and in serum-free medium. In addition its effect was markedly prolonged by a variety of other growth factors including insulin, platelet derived growth factor and fibroblast growth factor [19]. Like other cells responsive to bombesin, the effects on Swiss 3T3 cells were correlated with the ability of bombesin to bind to specific high affinity cell surface receptors which are distinct from those for other mitogens. A surface protein with an apparent molecular weight of 57 000–80 000 has been identified by chemical cross linking as a component of the bombesin receptor in these cells [19].

Following binding of BN/GRP to its receptor on these 3T3 cells, a series of events occur with mobilisation of calcium from the intracellular store which leads to a transient increase in cytosolic calcium and calcium efflux [19]. In addition transmodulation of EGF receptor affinity occurs, and an increased expression of both c-*myc* and c-*fos* oncogenes is detected. These data suggest that BN/GRP are important peptides in the regulation of cellular proliferation, 3T3 cells providing a model system for further elucidation of these events.

The mitogenic effects of BN/GRP have also been evaluated in a variety of human tumour cell lines including small cell lung cancer and non-small cell lung cancer. These studies were carried out because of the demonstration that many SCLC cell lines express high levels of BN/BLI. In addition high affinity binding receptors for BN/GRP have also been demonstrated in these tumour cell lines. Using a soft agarose clonogenic assay the influence of bombesin and GRP on the growth of these cell lines was tested. Studies were carried out in both serum supplemented medium and serum free medium. Bombesin and GRP were shown to be potent mitogens of SCLC growth with a peak effect observed at a concentration of added bombesin of 50 nM. A 70 to 150-fold stimulation of colony growth was observed in nine of ten SCLC cell lines grown in serum free medium. However, no effect of bombesin was observed in serum supplemented medium. No growth stimulation by bombesin was observed in cell lines originating from non-small cell lung cancer, malignant melanoma and from kidney tumours [20].

Although high affinity binding receptors for bombesin have been identified in approximately 30% of SCLC lines, there is no obvious correlation between the mitogenic effects of bombesin and the presence or absence of these receptors. In addition there is no obvious correlation between the amount of bombesin expressed by these cell lines and their response to exogenous added bombesin. These data suggest that in SCLC the mitogenic effect of bombesin and/or GRP may be mediated through mechanisms other than binding to receptors, i.e., through stimulation of the release of other exogenous hormones by the tumour, such as insulin or glucagon or through activation of other gene products.

Other explanations for the lack of correlation between the response to bombesin and the number of receptors detected include peptide mediated receptor down-regulation which is related to the constant release of bombesin into the culture medium. Thus, in isolated pancreatic acini pre-incubation of cells with bombesin, desensitisation of enzyme secretion is induced by reducing the number of active receptors available to interact with bombesin and stimulate secretion. Receptor down-regulation has been investigated in SCLC with GRP 1–27 and GRP 14–17. The results with GRP were almost identical to those obtained with bombesin. Moreover, the mitogenicity of GRP was clearly demonstrated to be a property of the terminal portion of the 27 amino acid peptide and little or no mitogenic effect was observed with the proximal peptide fragment (GRP 1–6). In contrast, analogues of bombesin with poor affinity binding for bombesin receptors had little or no effect on the clonal growth of SCLC tumour cells. These results with bombesin and GRP using a soft agarose clonogenic assay have confirmed the mitogenic effect of these peptides for SCLC growth. Weber et al., using an alternative assay to the clonogenic assay, have also confirmed these mitogenic effects in SCLC [22].

These data suggest that bombesin and GRP are important growth factors for SCLC. The finding of significant concentrations of these peptides in SCLC tumours and the identification of high affinity binding receptors for bombesin on these cells suggest that bombesin and GRP may function as autocrine growth factors. To test this hypothesis further the effect of monoclonal antibodies to bombesin on the growth of SCLC cells both in vivo and in vitro has been investigated. A monoclonal antibody (211) which binds the carboxy-terminal region of bombesin like peptides has been demonstrated to inhibit markedly the growth of SCLC cells both in vitro and also in vivo when injected subcutaneously into athymic nude mice. This antibody (211) blocks bombesin interaction with its receptor in a dose related fashion, and at high concentrations almost completely inhibits the binding of bombesin to its high affinity receptor [21].

These data further confirm that in SCLC cells BN/GRP has an important physiological role and may function as autocrine growth factor. Preliminary clinical investigation have been carried out on a small number of patients with SCLC who have been treated with a dosage of 1 mg/m^2 of this antibody. At these dose levels there have been no responses. In these patients, throughout the month of therapy, serum levels of mouse anti-211 antibody were detectable. One patient developed an anti-idiotype antibody response three weeks after the cessation of therapy. Further studies are required to determine if modulation of bombesin receptor interaction *in vivo* will have an important role in controlling growth of these tumour cells [24].

The finding of abundant BLI positive cells in a normal bronchial mucosa has also stimulated investigators to identify the effect of these peptides on normal bronchial epithelium [23]. Willey *et al.* have assessed the mitogenic effects of bombesin and GRP on human bronchial epithelium growth in the presence or absence of epidermal growth factor. Bombesin and GRP increased the colony forming efficiency and clonal growth of these normal human bronchial cells. These effects were seen both in the presence and absence of EGF and the addition of EGF did not cause any appreciable increase in clonal growth above that observed with either peptide alone. Thus as has been shown for SCLC, BN/GRP are potent mitogens for the growth of normal human bronchial epithelial cells and may play an important physiological regulatory role. Supporting data for this hypothesis has come from the demonstration that in infants with respiratory distress syndrome there is a relative paucity of bronchial BLI positive cells. All of the above data confirm that in addition to their many physiological effects bombesin and GRP are important mitogens for cellular growth. Clearly a greater understanding of their interaction with the receptor and how they may influence the growth of both normal and malignant cells would be of importance in the design of alternative therapies for the control of malignant growth.

CONCLUSIONS

In recent years, we have begun to understand the physiological function of BN/GRP, and its role in human malignancy. The recent elucidation of the molecular biology of BN/GRP perhaps could lead to the development of new alternatives for treating cancers in patients in whom such peptides have been demonstrated to be important in the maintenance of cell proliferation.

REFERENCES

1 Anastasia, A., Erspamer, V. and Bucci, M. Isolation and structure of bombesin and alytesin, two analogous active peptides from the skin of the European amphibians Bombina and Alytes. *Experientia (Basel).* 1971, **27**: 166–167.

2 Walsh, J.H., Wong, H.C. and Dockray, G.J. Bombesin-like peptides in mammals. *Fed Proc.* 1978, **38**: 2315–2319.
3 McDonald, T.J., Nilsson, G., Vagne, M., Ghatei, M., Bloom, S.R. and Mutt V. A gastrin releasing peptide from the porcine non-antral gastric tissue. *Gut.* 1978, **19**: 767–774.
4 Panula, P. Histochemistry and function of bombesin-like peptides. *Med Biol.* 1986, **64**: 177–192.
5 Wharton, J., Polak, J.M., Bloom, S.R., Ghatei, M.A., Solcia, E., Brown, M.R. and Pearse, A.G.E. Bombesin-like immunoreactivity in the lung. *Nature.* 1978, **273**: 769–770.
6 Cutz, E., Chan, W. and Track, N. Bombesin, calcitonin and leu-enkephalin in endocrine cells of human lung. *Experientia (Basel).* 1981, **37**: 765–767.
7 Naylor, S.L., Sakaguchi, A.Y., Spindel, E. and Chin, W.W. Human gastrin-releasing peptide gene is located on chromosome 18[1]. *Somatic Cell Mol Genet.* 1987, **13(1)**: 87–91.
8 Lebacq-Verheyden, A.M., Bertness, V., Kirsch, I., Hollis, G.F., McBride, O.W. and Battey, J. Human gastrin releasing peptide gene maps to chromosome 18. *Somatic Cell Mol Genet.* 1987, **13(1)**: 81–86.
9 Sausville, E.A., Lebacq-Verheyden, A.M., Spindel, E.R., Cuttitta, F., Gazdar, A.F. and Battey, J.F. Expression of the gastrin-releasing peptide gene in human small cell lung cancer. *J Biol Chem.* 1986, **261**: 2451–2457.
10 Cuttitta, F., Fedorko, J., Gu, J., Sausville, E., Lebacq-Verheyden, A.M., Linnoila, R.I., Mulshine, J.L. and Battey, J.F. Gastrin releasing peptide gene associated peptides (GGAPs) are expressed in normal human fetal lung and small cell lung cancer. *Regul Pept.* 1987, **19**: 105 (Abstr).
11 Spindel, E.R., Chin, W.W., Price, J., Rees, L.H., Besser, G.M. and Habener, J.F. Cloning and characterisation of cDNAs encoding human gastrin-releasing peptide. *Proc Natl Acad Sci USA.* 1984, **81**: 5699–5703.
12 Jensen, S., Cuttitta, F., Winton, T., Patterson, G.A., Chamberlain, D., Ihde D. and Linnoila I. Concordant expression of gastrin releasing releasing peptide (GRP) and GRP gene associated peptides (GCAPs) in primary and metastatic human small cell lung cancers (SCLSs): an immunohistochemical analysis. *Regul Pept.* 1987, **19**: 116 (Abstr).
13 Hamid, Q., Springall, D.R., Giaid, A. *et al.* The expression of human pro-bombesin gene in small cell carcinoma of the lung. *In situ* hybridisation with cRNA probe. *Regul Pept.* 1987, **19**: 113 (Abstr).
14 Berridge, M.J. and Irvine, R.R. Inositol triphosphate, a novel second messenger in cellular signal transduction. *Nature.* 1984, **312**: 315–321.
15 Takuwa, N., Takuwa, U., Bollag, W.E. and Rasmussen, H. The effects of bombesin on polyphosphoinositide and calcium metabolism in Swiss 3T3 cells. *J Biol Chem.* 1987, **262**: 182–188.
16 Wakelam, M.J., Davies, S.A., Houslay, M.D., McKay, I., Marshall, C.J. and Hall, A. Normal p21 N-ras couples bombesin and other growth factor receptors to inositol phosphate production. *Nature.* 1986, **323**: 173–176.
17 Trepel, J.B., Moyer, J., Heikkilla, R., Neckers, L.M. and Sausville, E.A. Second messengers of bombesin action in human small cell lung cancer. *Regul Pept.* 1987, **19**: 141 (Abstr).

18 Rozengurt, E. and Sinnett-Smith, J. Bombesin stimulation of DNA synthesis and cell division in cultures of Swiss 3T3 cells. *Proc Natl Acad Sci USA*. 1983, **80**: 2936–2940.

19 Rozengurt, E.A., Zachary, I., Sinnett-Smith, J. and Nanberg, E. Early events elicited by bombesin and other growth factors in quiescent Swiss 3T3 cells. *Regul Pept*. 1987, **19**: 136 (Abstr).

20 Carney, D.N., Cuttitta, F., Moody, T.W. and Minna, J.D. Selective stimulation of small lung cancer clonal growth by bombesin and gastrin-releasing peptide. *Cancer Res*. 1987, **47**: 821–825.

21 Cuttitta, F., Carney, D.N., Mulshine, J., Moody, T.W., Fedorko, J., Fischler, A. and Minna, J.D. Bombesin-like peptides can function as autocrine growth factors in human small cell lung cancer. *Nature*. 1985, **316**: 823–826.

22 Weber, S., Zuckerman, J.E., Bostwick, D.G., Bensch, K.G., Sikic, B.I. and Raffin, T.A. Gastrin releasing peptide is a selective mitogen for small cell lung carcinoma *in vitro*. *J Clin Invest*. 1985, **75**: 306–309.

23 Willey, J.C., Lechner, J.F. and Harris, C.C. Bombesin and the C-terminal tetradecapeptide of gastrin-releasing peptide are growth factors for normal human bronchial epithelial cells. *Exp Cell Res*. 1984, **153**: 245–248.

24 Mulshine, J.L., Cuttitta, F., Ingallil, A. *et al.* Immunologic blockade of autocrine stimulation of lung cancer by gastrin releasing peptide (GRP). A new therapeutic approach. *Regul Pept*. 1987, **19**: 129. (Abstr).

5 HUMAN RETROVIRUSES AND MALIGNANCY

A.G. DALGLEISH

R ETROVIRUSES are a single taxonomic group of RNA viruses which replicate through a host cell intermediate by encoding RNA directed DNA polymerase (reverse transcriptase). Upon infection reverse transcriptase catalyses the synthesis of a double stranded intermediate, the provirus, from the single stranded virus RNA. The provirus subsequently becomes integrated into host chromosome DNA and serves as a template for viral genomic and messenger RNA transcription by the host cells RNA synthetic and processing systems (Fig. 5.1). Other features unique to retroviruses include a diploid RNA genome, a high frequency of intermolecular recombination between related viruses and the ability to acquire host genes termed oncogenes which encode functions responsible for neoplastic transformation.

Retroviruses occur in host vertebrate species where they are associated with a diversity of diseases which include malignancies such as carcinoma, sarcomas, lymphomas and leukaemia, as well as other haematological disorders such as anaemia and aplasia, wasting autoimmune disorders, arthritis and a variety of neurological conditions.

The first retroviruses were discovered in the early 1900s and the first retrovirus that was clearly shown to be the causative agent of a tumour was reported in 1911 by Peyton Rous [1]. The Rous sarcoma virus (RSV) has been one of the mose useful of the RNA tumour viruses and has been extensively studied with regards to its transformation properties and host susceptibility.

Retroviruses are divided into three major subfamilies mainly by their pathogenic properties *viz*: the oncovirinae; which include those with oncogenic potential, lentivirinae; including the prototype visna virus of sheep which cause slow, progressive degeneration of the central nervous system and the spumavirinae or foamy viruses; which are not known to the pathogenic. Endogenous viruses which pass vertically in the germ line are included within the oncovirinae which are further sub-classified on the basis of virion morphology, as defined by electron microscopy.

Most retroviruses carry three genes in the order 5' *gag, pol, env,* 3' where *gag* encodes a precurser protein which is cleaved to yield three or four internal structural proteins, *pol* encodes reverse transcriptase, and *env* encodes the envelope proteins at least one of which is glycosylated. The genome is capped by long terminal repeats (LTRs) at both ends which are responsible for the integration of the DNA provirus with cellular DNA and contain promotor and enhancer sequences of viral gene expression.

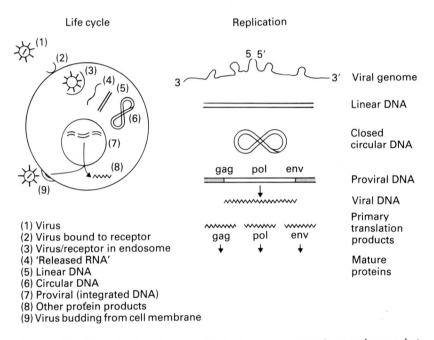

(1) Virus
(2) Virus bound to receptor
(3) Virus/receptor in endosome
(4) 'Released RNA'
(5) Linear DNA
(6) Circular DNA
(7) Proviral (integrated DNA)
(8) Other protein products
(9) Virus budding from cell membrane

Fig. 5.1   The life cycle of a retrovirus. Most retroviruses enter via an endosome, but some, such as HIV fuse directly at the surface.

Other genes may be inserted between the LTRs by recombination such as the insertion of a cellular oncogene sequence or alternative genetic sequences such as those seen in bovine leukaemia virus (BLV) and the visna virus of sheep. These both have additional functional genes which are not oncogenes, as they have no cellular gene homology. However, these genes are capable of acting on cellular genes, as well as on their own reproductive control gene, at a considerable distance, and hence they are known as trans-activating genes as opposed to *cis* genes which only act on immediate neighbouring genes.

MECHANISMS OF ONCOGENICITY

Retroviruses can cause neoplasia either acutely or chronically. RSV causes tumours in chickens within a few days of infection as do other retroviruses in other hosts. These viruses transform target cells by carrying specific transforming sequences called *onc* genes. The viral genes (v-*onc*) which cause transformation are derived from cellular (c-*onc*) genes that apparently exert their oncogenic effect when combined into the viral genome by strong promotor signals in the proviral LTR. Viral *onc* genes are not necessary for replication and in most cases acquisition of an *onc* gene sacrifices viral genes required for replication. They can only be grown in association with replication competent viruses although it should be stressed that RSV is an exception to this rule.

It is now known that the cellular sequences from which these viral *onc* genes are derived, are involved in growth and differentiation control in the normal cell and it does not seem too surprising that a gene positively controlling growth should lead to cancer when allowed to express outside of its regulatory genes. However, although acutely oncogenic viruses have been studied more intensively than other retroviruses they are only rarely or sporadically found in nature which suggests that each isolate represents a recombinant virus. They are not transmitted from one host to another, either because they are defective or because they are so rapidly pathogenic that there is a strong selection against natural persistence by transmission. 'Slow' neoplasms on the other hand are commonly seen in nature. The slowness or chronic nature refers to the long latent period between infection and the appearance of clinical disease which may well present as a fast growing and highly malignant tumour. The animals are usually chronically viraemic prior to the appearance of a tumour which may be induced by a multistage process. Details will not be given here except to mention that some slow viruses integrate near or next to cellular oncogenes and by a variety of mechanisms enhance their expression.

Other viruses already mentioned notably BLV and visna as well as all the human retroviruses isolated so far contain trans-activating genes. These may act on cellular genes which are not in close proximity to the virus. These genes may not necessarily be cellular oncogenes and detailed study should give valuable insights into the disorders in cellular gene control which lead to cancer expression [2, 3]. Indeed interference with negative regulators of cellular oncogenes: anti-oncogenes, may yet be shown to be one of the major mechanisms of induction of oncogenesis.

HUMAN RETROVIRUSES

Against a background of numerous retroviruses causing a variety of diseases most with readily recognisable human counterparts in numerous animal species, it is not surprising that a large scale search for retroviruses associated with human disease has been undertaken.

What is surprising is that with the exception of numerous dubious isolates [2, 3] the search was so disappointingly negative that it was largely abandoned by most investigators long before the isolation of the first real human retrovirus to be associated with disease was discovered by Robert Gallo and his colleagues of the NIH, Bethesda, USA in 1978 and reported in 1980 [4]. This virus was called the human T cell leukaemia/lymphoma virus type 1 (HTLV1).

HTLV1

Two lines of enquiry led to the discovery of the first human T cell lymphotropic virus. One was the belief that such viruses existed and therefore new methods of isolation and detection would need to be employed to detect them and secondly the recognition of the high incidence of a T cell malignancy termed adult T cell leukaemia/lymphoma (ATLL), in southern Japan [5]. The marked clustering of ATLL and its distinct clinical features strongly suggested a viral aetiology. As C type particles had already been reported in patients with T cell lymphomas the viral hypothesis was tested by looking for antibodies in the serum of ATLL patients against an established cell line from one such patient. All patients with ATLL had antibodies against cytoplasmic antigens in a T cell line (MT-1) as did 26% of healthy adults living in the endemic area, as opposed to only 2% in non-endemic areas. However, only after HTLV1 had been isolated by Gallo and colleagues [4] and the association with patients with ATLL established, were similar particles reported in MT-1 on electron microscopy. The virus was, therefore, presumed to be aetiologically linked to ATLL and, therefore, called the adult T cell leukaemia virus (ATLV).

The infectivity of this virus was established in co-cultivation experiments with fresh cord cells which could be immortalised by ATLV [6]. Prior to this, Gallo and his co-workers had been working on the theory that human retroviral particles were too few to be detected by electron microscopy and, therefore, attempted to refine the reverse transcriptase. In order to demonstrate their origin unequivocally (since they could have been unusual cellular polymerases detectable because their number was increased in diseased cells) a much larger number of the putative viruses were required.

Human cell lines are difficult to grow in the laboratory and it therefore seemed logical to look for a growth factor that would allow for the proliferation of particular lymphocytes on the grounds that the number of virions may also, therefore, be increased. In 1976 Gallo and his colleagues discovered a growth factor specific for mature T cells called the T cell growth factor, TCGF or interleukin 2 [7] which allowed for the selective growth of T lymphocyte populations *in vitro*. The stage was then set for the first isolation of a human T cell retrovirus which was achieved in 1978 [4]. This was obtained from cultured T lymphocytes from a patient with a skin T cell lymphoma termed mycosis fungoides. A second isolate was obtained from a patient with Sezary's syndrome.

Detailed characterisation of the virus followed which showed that the retrovirus was magnesium-dependent and not manganese as in most animal retroviruses. In addition the isolation of specific monoclonal antibodies and nucleic acid probes was achieved. The cells from which HTLV1 was isolated were OKT4 lymphocytes, the same subtype as the tumour cells of ATL. As no definitive serological data had been obtained in the USA to link HTLV1 with a specific disease, coded sera provided by Y. Ito, N. Nakao, T. Aoki and their colleagues were examined in Gallo's laboratory, which showed almost 100% of the sera of ATL patients to be positive. Subsequent studies were to show that both isolates were the same virus and that all subsequent isolates from the USA, Japan and the UK represented the same serotype.

The clinical features of ATLL were first recognised as a distinct clinical entity in the West by Catovsky and his colleagues at the Hammersmith Hospital in London, who described the occurrence of ATLL in Caribbean immigrants to the UK [8]. This directed attention to the Caribbean as the second endemic HTLV1 area after Japan. In the light of later findings it now seems likely that the American patients from whom the first isolates were obtained suffered from ATLL with predominant skin involvement. The clinical features include hypercalcaemia with or without bone lesions as well as hepatosplenomegaly and lymphadenopathy, features which are characteristic of sarcoidosis. This is also prominent in the Caribbean area as well as in Negroes in south east USA. This raises the possibility that sarcoidosis could be due to a similar agent [9] although no retrovirus has yet been shown to be associated with sarcoidosis.

Epidemiology of HTLV1

HTLV1 has now been shown to be endemic in the south east of the USA, parts of South America, parts of southern Italy, the Arctic, the American Indians and Canadian immigrants to Cayenne as well as many parts of Africa. The virus has also been detected in the Surinam population of Holland, as well as in populations at risk from AIDS. It has also been found in association with T cell malignancies in Caucasian people living in the UK [2, 3, 10].

HTLV1 as the causative agent of ATLL

The aetiological association of HTLV1 with ATLL is based on the following observations: firstly, geographically, the areas of high incidence of ATLL correspond closely with those of high prevalence of HTLV1 infection as adduced from seroepidemiological surveys. Secondly, all individuals with ATLL have evidence of HTLV1 infection. Thirdly, the ATLL tumour cells carry HTLV1 proviruses whereas non-malignant cells from the same patients are not necessarily infected. Fourthly, HTLV1 transforms human and animal T cells *in vitro* and finally, HTLV1 is closely related to simian retroviruses which are oncogenic in experimental animals [2]. In addition, seroepidemiological studies suggest that only about one in 80 infected people develop ATLL and that it may take several decades to do so. This data suggests that a co-factor or a 'second hit' is necessary for malignancy to develop. The mechanisms whereby HTLV1 infection leads to malignancy will be discussed in further detail at the end of the chapter.

HTLV2

The first isolate of HTLV2 was from a patient with T cell variant hairy cell leukaemia [11]. Although subsequent studies have failed to link HTLV2 to hairy cell leukaemia [10], a second isolate of HTLV2 has recently been reported from a patient with atypical hairy cell leukaemia, as well as antibodies to HTLV2 in a patient with a 'new' T cell lymphoproliferative disease [12] which suggests a possible causal role in some T cell malignancies. Two other isolates of HTLV2 have been obtained from a New York drug addict with AIDS and a haemophiliac who did not have evidence of malignancy. The epidemiology of HTLV2 has not been thoroughly studied although it has been reported in London drug addicts. The increasing association with malignancy is in keeping with the ability of HTLV2, like HTLV1, to transform human lymphocytes *in vitro*. In spite of the paucity of isolates and seroepidemiology, HTLV2 is very similar to HTLV1 in both genomic structure as well as functionally and, therefore, future associations with T cell malignancies should not be surprising.

HTLV5

Recently, a new human retrovirus named HTLV5 has been isolated from a cutaneous T cell lymphoma. It is similar but distinct from HTLV1 and HTLV2 [13]. Further characterisation is needed to support these claims however.

AIDS and HIV

In spite of HTLV1 and 2, human retroviruses would probably have remained in comparative obscurity if it had not been for the sudden emergence of the acquired immunodeficiency syndrome (AIDS). Although it was first recognised as a distinct disease entity in early 1981, with hindsight it probably did not exist outside Africa until 1978 when the first cases presented in the USA and Haiti. AIDS was first recognised due to the occurrence of pneumocystitis carinii and Kaposi's sarcoma (KS) in previously healthy young homosexual men and reported to the Centre for Disease Control (CDC) in 1981. Both conditions were extremely rare outside immunosuppressed populations, such as patients with renal transplants, although a relatively benign form of KS manifesting on the lower limbs is not uncommon in older men of Mediterranean extraction.

It rapidly became clear that AIDS was endemic in American homosexuals, drug addicts and people from Haiti who manifested many and varied opportunistic infections as well as immunoblastic lymphomas, in addition to the early presentations described. Furthermore, it became apparent that many people in the AIDS at-risk categories were developing ominous signs of ill health such as persistent generalised lymphadenopathy and severe systemic symptoms such as weight loss, night sweats, diarrhoea, malaise, etc. which did not qualify for a diagnosis of AIDS (defined by the CDC as a reliably diagnosed disease indicative of cellular immune deficiency with no known underlying cause). Any doubt that the sudden emergence of these conditions in three well defined groups was due to an infectious agent was quickly dispelled with the recognition that AIDS was spreading through blood and its products such as factors VIII and IX used to treat haemophiliacs.

As the exponential rise in the number of AIDS cases continued a search for a likely candidate ensued. A new retrovirus was an attractive idea as many animal retroviruses cause immunodeficiency and allied diseases. For instance, Friend virus and avian leukosis viruses cause wasting syndromes in rats and birds respectively, equine infectious anaemia virus induces multiple immunopathies and Mason–Pfizer monkey virus has also been associated with immunodeficiency [2]. However, it was the feline leukaemia viruses of cats which cause leukaemia/lymphomas in some cats (reminiscent of HTLV1-induced disease in humans), and T cell depletion and opportunistic infections in others, that suggested that a virus similar to HTLV1, and therefore, a retrovirus might be the cause of AIDS [14].

Although HTLV1 is occasionally associated it is not the cause of AIDS. Indeed, the first isolation of a new human virus subsequently shown to be the causal agent of AIDS was reported in 1983 by Montagnier and his colleagues at the Pasteur Institute [15], who detected reverse transcriptase and cytopathic activity as well as viral particles on electronmicroscopy in PHA and interleukin 2 (IL2) stimulated cultured lymphocytes from a patient with lymphadenopathy. They noted the similarities of the new isolate to HTLV and suggested the term T lymphotrophic retrovirus whilst naming the virus LAV1 (lymphadenopathy virus). Other similar cultures followed and the causal association of LAV and AIDS remained obscure until Popovic and Gallo reported 48 isolations from AIDS and at-risk patients of a new retrovirus which they termed human T cell lymphotrophic virus type 3 (HTLV3). This was 'caught' in a virus producing cell line, thus enabling characterisation and the causal link with AIDS and related conditions to be established [16].

Subsequent studies have shown HTLV3 and LAV to be virtually identical. Levy and his colleagues from San Francisco have reported the isolation of similar viruses which they term AIDS related viruses (ARV) which, although they are similar to the LAV and HTLV3 isolates, are clearly more distant and furthermore have markedly different neutralisation properties [17]. In view of the growing terminology, an international committee has decided that all the different isolates should be termed human immunodeficiency viruses (HIV).

Simian AIDS (SAIDS) and the new African isolates

SAIDS was first recognised in 1983 at both the New England and Californian primate centers. D type retroviruses were initially isolated from the afflicted colonies although the similarity of these viruses to HTLV3 has led them to be termed STLV3 or simian immunodeficiency viruses (SIV). Serological studies have shown that STLV3 is present in approximately 50% of African green monkeys, but not in chimpanzees, baboons or colobus monkeys. African green vervets infected with STLV3 do not become ill, however, unlike macaques which manifest overt SAIDS following infection. These observations led to Africa as a possible origin of the AIDS virus. Serological screening studies in West Africa (where AIDS is not endemic) showed that antibodies to STLV3 were detected in healthy Senagalese prostitutes. This led to the isolation of a new virus distinct antigenically from other HIV isolates. Unfortunately it has since been shown to be a laboratory contaminant of SIV, which does not however detract from the importance of the above serological findings.

Another new isolate has been made by the Pasteur team and called LAV2. They noticed that some West African AIDS patients were repeatedly negative for serum antibodies to HIV. A virus similar yet distinct from HIV1, LAV2, was isolated from three patients. LAV2 does not appear to be associated with malignancy at the present time [18,19].

AIDS and cancer

HIV infection is associated with KS and malignant B cell lymphomas. Other cancers such as oro-pharyngeal and peri-rectal carcinomas as well as small cell cancers are being reported in at-risk populations who are not necessarily HIV seropositive. Most of these cancers may be due to oncogenic virus expression in an immunosuppressed state such as Epstein–Barr virus (EBV) and HTLV1 associated lymphomas, and papillomaviruses associated with squamous cell carcinomas. However, the sequence of events may not be as simple in all cases.

Kaposi's sarcoma

KS is a histological and clinical enigma, and its classification as a malignancy remains extremely controversial. It was discovered by

Moritz Kaposi over 100 years ago. It was noticed to affect men of Eastern European origin manifesting as a relatively benign condition consisting of purplish macules or nodules affecting the extremeties. In the late 1950s, an endemic form was described in Eastern and Central Africa that displayed four distinct clinical types namely: (a) locally indolent lesions with red-purple skin nodules with intact skin, (b) florid, locally invasive aggressive and fungating nodules; (c) disseminated mucocutaneous form, diffusely infiltrating the skin and deeper structures and which involves the underlying bone, and (d) a disseminated form with visceral disease including lymph node and lung involvement. Each type of KS may be subdivided into A or B depending upon the presence (A) or absence (B) of systemic symptoms. A simple classification recognises the endemic (or classical) indolent form seen in elderly East European men, African children in Equatorial Africa and transplant recipients, and secondly the aggressive epidemic form associated with HIV infection (AIDS). Histopathologically a wide variety of features are seen which suggests a multipotential mesenchymal cell of origin. Essentially vascular proliferations and spindle shaped neoplastic cells form in a network of reticular fibres which appear to be of an endothelial origin. Subclassifications are described which will not be discussed further. It does not appear to be an aneuploid monoclonal malignancy *per se.*

KS is known to occur in immunosuppressed patients such as post-transplant patients, where not only is it surprisingly uncommon but may regress upon withdrawal of immunosuppression. This makes a viral origin attractive. However, earlier studies linking cytomegalovirus to KS by Giraldo and associates in 1972 have not withstood detailed investigation. Indeed, the only clear viral link with KS appears to be HIV where the manifestation of KS commands a diagnosis of AIDS. However, KS seen in AIDS patients is different from the endemic or classical form in that it is aggressive, relatively refractory to treatment, involves the internal organs and may lead to death by strangulation, obstruction or haemorrhage within 6 months [9,10]. The occurrence of a new epidemic form of aggressive KS in Africa led us to look for the presence of HIV antibodies. Patients with HIV seroantibodies were more likely to have the aggressive as opposed to the endemic form of KS in Africa [15, 20].

Studies on KS tissues looking for viral integration have failed to describe an association with a number of candidate viruses which include CMV (cytomegalovirus), EBV, HTLV1, HTLV2, and papilloma viruses as well as many others (R.C. Gallo, personal communication). Moreover, even in HIV seropositive KS patients there is no evidence for HIV integration into KS at the molecular level. So what is the cause of this enigma and what is the mechanism of its HIV association? Obviously a hitherto uncharacterised virus is an attractive proposition and has been sought unsuccessfully by many workers. Indeed I and others have isolated HIV virus from supposedly HIV seronegative patients only to find the patients later seroconverted. Perhaps the most exciting work on KS at present is being undertaken by S.Z. Salahuddin in Robert Gallo's laboratory. Salahuddin has shown that an HTLV2 producing cell line produces a growth factor which allows KS to be grown *in vitro*. Furthermore, Salahuddin has been able to grow KS tissue in nude mice and preliminary studies indicate that KS cells produce an autologous growth factor which appears to be different from that produced by the HTLV2 cell line (personal communication).

It is possible that no discovered or undiscovered virus is associated with KS. Angiogenic substances could provoke endothelial proliferation and tumour proliferation. Tumour angiogenesis factor, heparin, prostaglandins, interleukin 1 and immune interferon are all capable of this function. Indeed the production of angiogenic lymphomas and T cell abnormalities are thought to be responsible for angioimmunoblastic lymphadenopathy, a condition which shares some features with AIDS. T cells appear to be increasingly implicated in a variety of regulatory functions [10] including endothelial cells and it is possible that HIV could destroy a subset of helper lymphocytes which specifically control endothelial cell function. Non-HIV associated KS may be associated with excessive paracrine angiogenic lymphokines in response to an external agent or agents.

Lymphomas

The association of B cell non-Hodgkin's lymphoma (NHL) in patients with AIDS and pre-AIDS is well established [21]. Although Hodgkin's disease (HD) is not uncommon in the AIDS at-risk age group, there is increasing evidence to suggest that there might be a real increase in the incidence of HD in HIV infected people. Those patients with HIV and NHL respond poorly to therapy, have a high recurrence rate and a prediliction for opportunistic infection. Furthermore, many (<25%) HIV infected patients with NHL also have KS. NHLs in AIDS is similar to that observed in association with iatrogenic immunosuppression such as in transplant patients. Both have been observed to evolve from polyclonal to monoclonal B cell proliferation. Oncogenic viruses such as EBV may cause B cell proliferation which, against a background of immunosuppression, may allow a second 'event' or mutation to occur leading to malignancy. However, an increasing number of HIV positive NHL cases have been reported as being negative for EBV. Many are positive for HTLV1 however, which may coexist with HIV in up to 10% of cases. Perhaps other oncogenic viruses exist which have not yet been discovered. A possible example is the new human B lymphotropic virus isolated from patients with HIV and NHLs reported by Salahuddin and Gallo [22]. Further characterisation and information on its role in lymphoma pathogenesis remains eagerly awaited.

It also remains possible that HIV could itself be oncogenic, in a similar way to animal retroviruses which have been previously described. Although there is no direct evidence to support this contention, molecular characterisation of HIV continues to find new genes, new methods of gene regulation and new possibilities for interaction with cellular genes, and, therefore, this hypothesis cannot be ignored completely. However, it is more likely that HIV acts as an initiator and other viruses act as promotors in the induction of malignancy [2, 3, 9, 23].

MECHANISMS OF HTLV AND HIV PATHOGENESIS

HTLV1 causes ATL in only 1–2% of people infected with a latency period of up to 30 years. How does it do this? One of the most remarkable features of human retroviruses is the ability to reproduce the pathogenic effects *in vitro* in a much reduced time period.

HTLV1 causes infected cells to increase the number of interleukin 2 receptors as defined by the Tac monoclonal antibody. This correlates with increased Tac expression seen *in vivo*. Furthermore, HTLV1 is also capable of immortalising T cells in much the same way as EBV immortalises B cells, but by what mechanism? Unlike the acute and chronic retrovirusus described above, HTLV1 and HTLV2 have an extra gene which has been called the 'X' lor, or 'tat' gene by different workers and at different times. The tat gene is inserted between the *env* gene and the 3'LTR (Fig. 5.2), which is similar to the oncogene site in RSV. 'Tat' is not an oncogene, however, in that it is not homologous to any cellular sequences. It is capable of regulating production of HTLV1 by influencing the 5′LTR. Perhaps more importantly it has been shown to transactivate not only IL-2 but also its receptor [18,24]. HTLV1 does not integrate at any conserved site in the host cell DNA so it is unlikely to act like a chronic virus by influencing cellular oncogenes in *cis*. However, by turning on IL-2 and its receptor it is activating the infected lymphocyte in such a way that it may autologously stimulate itself. HTLV1 malignant cells are however IL-2 independent and moreover they are monoclonal. It therefore seems likely that HTLV1 initiates chronic proliferation thereby making the occurrence of a second promotor event leading to monoclonal malignancy more likely. The nature of this second event is unknown although ATL appears to be associated with abnormalities of the 14th chromosome. An uncorrected chance genetic translocation therefore remains a possibility.

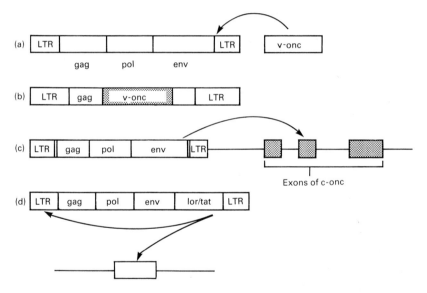

Fig. 5.2   Different mechanisms whereby retroviruses cause malignancy (a) structure of retrovirus; (b) replication defective oncogene bearing virus; (c) *cis* acting virus 'turning on' a cellular oncogene; (d) retrovirus containing transactivator gene.

Little is known about HTLV2 except that *in vitro* it behaves like HTLV1, although it is less efficient at immortalisation. This may explain the limited association with malignancy *in vivo*. It is also able to turn on IL-2 and its receptor by transactivation of these cellular genes by the HTLV2 *tat* gene. Overall, HTLV1 and HTLV2 share a 60% homology at the nucleic acid sequence level.

MOLECULAR BIOLOGY OF HIV

In addition to the *gag, pol, env* genes, HIV contains at least another five genes, namely *sor* (short open reading frame), 3'*orf* (open reading frame), *tat, art/trs* which also relate transactivating functions, and a new gene R (Fig. 5.3). At present, little is known about the functions of *sor* and 3'*orf* products. Whereas experiments with deletion mutants in the 3'*orf* region suggest that 3'*orf* is not required for replication or cytopathogenicity, they also suggest that the two are not necessarily coupled. The role of *sor* is controversial as Sodroski and co-workers [25] have found the *sor* gene unnecessary for the replication of cytopathic effects of HIV and Fisher *et al.* from Gallo's laboratory (personal communication) have found that *sor* is extremely important in contributing to the infectivity of HIV.

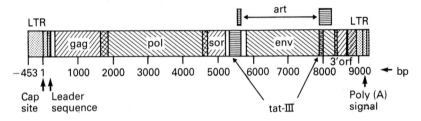

Fig. 5.3 The genetic structure and proteins of HIV. Two genes have recently been described, whose function has yet to be elucidated.

In contrast to the uncertainties of *sor* and *orf* 3' the functions of *tat* and *art/trs* are clearly defined. Viruses defective in *tat* and *art/trs* do not replicate *in vitro* or induce cytopathic effects. Both *tat* and *art/trs* encode transactivating functions, i.e. the products of these genes act upon other HIV genes to stimulate their expression. *Tat* is required for high level expression, and is encoded by two exons. The doubly spliced message probably encodes an 86 amino acid protein with structural features similar to those of nucleic acid binding proteins. The *tat*III gene product results in an increase in protein syntheseis without a comparable rise in the steady state level of mRNAs as a consequence of the elevation of LTR directed gene expression.

This lack of effect of *tat*III on viral mRNA concentration and the presence on the 5' side of viral mRNAs of nucleotide sequences which respond to *tat*III, initiated studies by Haseltine and co-workers [26] which showed that transactivation by *tat*III requires a post-translational step. Further mutation detection studies identified a new gene known as *art* (anti-repressor transactivator, also known as *trs* (trans acting regulator of splicing), the product of which (116 amino acids) allows translation of HIV *gag* and *env* mRNAs, thus unlocking a block imposed on viral expression. *Tat* and *art* (*trs*) gene products are clearly potent regulators of gene expression and are probably involved in the control of the latency and expression phases of the HIV life cycle [2, 3].

The cytopathogenic effect of HIV *in vitro* is limited to cells bearing the CD4 antigen which is clearly the receptor for HIV in human cells [27]. Indeed the interaction between the CD4 and envelope glyco-protein of HIV contributes considerably to the pathogenicity of HIV as the large fusion cells formed ultimately die.

There is considerable genetic diversity amongst the different iso-lates of HIV and relatively low levels of neutralising antibodies are elicited which when present show poor cross neutralisation activity with diverse isolates [17]. Indeed, the only constant features of cell HIV isolates including the newer LAV2 and SIV is that they bind to the CD4 antigen and that blocking with certain monoclonal antibodies to different epitopes of CD4 prevents infection. This remarkable prop-erty may prove to be the Achilles' heel of the virus as a CD4 anti-idiotype vaccine may be more effective than current envelope based vaccine approaches [28]. Unfortunately all current vaccine strategies have major theoretical and practical limitations and many eminent workers in the field feel that a vaccine against HIV may never be produced.

Conclusions

In spite of the enormous explosion in our knowledge of HIV over the last 2–3 years we are still not clear about how HIV causes cancer in infected individuals at a higher rate than can be reasonably accounted for by immunosuppression. As molecular studies continue to reveal new and tortuously complicated genetic control mechanisms in HIV it would not be unreasonable to suspect that HIV may be able to transactivate cellular genes or those of other putatively oncogenic viruses to allow expression of malignancy. The ability to destroy the conductor of the immunological orchestra, the CD4 lymphocyte, has allowed a hitherto uninvestigated scenario to develop and we may yet learn a great deal more about the immune system and cancer from this virus. Whatever the eventual outcome of AIDS and AIDS research, it would appear clear that lessons learnt from studying HIV and other retroviruses are going to produce incalculable benefits in our understanding of other diseases and in particular malignancy.

REFERENCES

1 Rous, P. A sarcoma of the fowl transmissable by an agent separable from tumour cells. *J Exp Med*. 1911, **13**: 397–411.
2 Weiss, R.A., Teich, N.M., Barmus, H.E. and Coffin, J. (eds) *RNA Tumour Viruses: Molecular Biology of Tumour Viruses*. 2nd ed. New York: Cold Spring Harbor (Monograph series), 1985.
3 Dalgleish, A.G. and Malkovsky, M. Advances in human retroviruses. In: Klein, G., (ed) *Adv Cancer Res*. London: Academic Press (in press).
4 Poeisz, B.J., Ruscetti, F.W., Gazdar, A.F., Bunn, P.A., Minna, J.D. and Gallo, R.C. Detection and isolation of type c retrovirus particles from fresh and cultured lymphocytes of a patient with cutaneous T cell lymphoma. *Proc Natl Acad Sci USA*. 1980, **77**: 7415–7419.
5 Uchijama, T., Yadoi, J., Sagaura, K., Takatsuki, K. and Uchinott. Adult T cell leukaemia. Clinical and haematological features of 16 cases. *Blood*. 1977, **50**: 481–492.
6 Hunsmann, G. and Hinuma, Y. Human adult T-cell leukaemia virus and its association with disease. In: Klein, G. (ed) *Advances in Viral Oncology*. New York: Raven Press, 1985, **5**: 147–172.
7 Morgan, D.A., Ruscetti, F.W. and Gallo, R.C. Selective growth of T-lymphocytes from normal human bone marrow. *Science*. 1976, **193**: 1007–1008.
8 Catovsky, D., Greaves, M.F., Rose, M. *et al*. Adult T cell lymphoma leukaemia in Blacks from the West Indies. *Lancet*. 1982, **i**: 639–643.
9 Dalgleish, A.G. Human retroviruses. *Aust NZ J Med*. 1985, **15**: 375–385.
10 Dalgleish, A.G. and Weiss, R.A. Human retroviruses. In: Zuckerman, Pattison and Banatvala (eds) *Clinical Virology*. Chichester and London: Wiley, 1986, 525–550.
11 Kalyanaraman, V.S., Sarngadharan, M.O., Robert-Guroff, M., Miyohi, I., Blayney, D., Golde, D., Gallo, R.C. A subtype of HTLV associated with a variant of hairy cell leukaemia. *Science*. 1982, **218**: 571–573.
12 Sohn, C.C., Blayney, D.W., Misset, J.L. *et al*. Leukopenic chronic T cell leukaemia mimicking hairy cell leukaemia: association with human retroviruses. *Blood*. 1986, **67**: 949–956.
13 Manzari, V., Gismondi, A., Barilliari *et al*. HTLV-V: A new human retrovirus isolated in a tac negative T cell leukaemia/lymphoma. *Science*. 1987, **238**: 1581–1583.
14 Hardy, W.D. Jr. Feline retroviruses. In: Klein, G. (ed) *Advances in Viral Oncology*. New York: Raven Press, 1985, **5**: 1–35.
15 Barré-Sinoussi, F., Chermon, J.C., Rey, F. *et al*. Isolation of T lymphotropic retroviruses from a patient at risk of AIDS. *Science*. 1983, **220**: 868–870.
16 Wong-Staal, F. and Gallo, R.C. Human T cell lymphotropic viruses. *Nature*. 1985, **317**: 395–403.
17 Weiss, R.A., Clapham, P.R., Weber, J.N., Dalgleish, A. G., Berman, P.W. and

Laskey, L.A. Variable and conserved neutralisation antigens of HIV. *Nature.* 1986, **342**: 572–575.

18 Clavel, F. HIV2 the West Africa AIDS virus. *AIDS.* 1987, **1**: 135–140.

19 Kanki, P.J. West African human retrovirus related to STLV-III. *AIDS.* 1987, **1**: 141–145.

20 Bayley, A.C., Downing, R.G., Chiengsong-Popov, R., Tedder, R.S., Dalgleish, A.G. and Weiss, R.A. HTLV-III serology distinguishes atypical and ludemic Kaposi's sarcoma in Africa. *Lancet.* 1985, **i**: 359–361.

21 Ziegler, J.L., Beckstead, J.A., Volberding, P. *et al.* New Hodgkin's lymphoma in 90 homosexual men. *New Eng J Med.* 1984, **311**: 565–570.

22 Salahuddin, S.Z., Ablashi, D., Markham, P.D. *et al.* Isolation of a new virus HBLV in patients with lymphoproliferative disorders. *Science.* 1986: **234**: 596–601.

23 Ziegler, J.L. and Levy, J.A. AIDS and cancer. In: Broder, S. (ed) *AIDS.* New York: Raven Press, 1986.

24 Greene, W., Leonard, W.J., Wano, Y. *et al.* Transactivator gene of HTLV induces IL-2 receptor and gene expression. *Science.* 1986, **232**: 877–880.

25 Sodroski, J., Goh, W.C., Rosen, C.A. *et al.* Replicative and cytopathic potential of HIV with sor gene deletions. *Science.* 1986, **231**: 1549–1553.

26 Sodroski, J., Goh, W.C., Rosen, C., Dayton, A., Terwilliger, T. and Haseltine, W.A. A second post transcriptional transactivation gene required for HTLV-III replication. *Nature.* 1986, **321**: 412–417.

27 Dalgleish, A.G., Beverley, P.C.L., Clapham, P., Crawford, D., Greaves, M. and Weiss, R.A. The CD4 (T4) antigen is an essential component of the receptor for the AIDS retrovirus. *Nature.* 1984, **312**: 763–767.

28 Dalgleish, A.G., Thomson, B.J., Chanh, T., Malkovsky, M., Kennedy, R.C. Neutralisation of HIV isolates by anti-idiopathic antibodies which mimic the CD4 epitope: a potential AIDS vaccine. *Lancet.* 1987, **ii**: 1047–1050.

6 RADIOLABELLED MONOCLONAL ANTIBODIES IN THE MANAGEMENT OF CANCER

G.B. SIVOLAPENKO, H. KALOFONOS AND
A.A. EPENETOS

THE CONCEPT of using specific agents for the diagnosis and therapy of diseases was one of the earliest goals of medicine and was imaginatively described as 'magic bullet' treatment by Paul Ehrlich. The first example of the use of antibodies against cancer was reported in 1895 by Hericourt and Richet who treated a human osteogenic sarcoma with antisera [1]. Tumour localisation, using radiolabelled antibody was first introduced by Pressman and Keighley in 1948 [2]. Since then, several workers have demonstrated both in experimental models and in clinical studies the potential value of radiolabelled tumour associated polyclonal antisera.

The development of the techniques of monoclonal antibody production has led to the synthesis of antibodies that recognise a wide range of antigenic determinants on the surface of human tumour cells. This has presented new opportunities for the study of experimental cancer and has a potential use in the diagnosis and treatment of cancer. Radiolabelled monoclonal antibodies have been shown to localise successfully to a wide range of tumours in experimental animals [3] and in patients [4]. Having successfully demonstrated antibody localisation it is a natural step to apply labelled antibodies for targeted radiotherapy. Clinical trials of this approach have, shown only limited success.

In order to improve upon existing results it is important to identify the reasons why antibody guided irradiation has, so far, only been of limited value. The therapeutic system which comes closest to the ideal is radioiodine treatment of thyroid carcinoma. In that system there is an active and very specific mechanism of radionuclide uptake with high target to non-target ratios. Levels of 0.1–1% of the administered dose can be achieved, with an effective half life of the radionuclide in the tumour, of between 58 and 100 hours.

Radiolabelled monoclonal antibody therapy needs to achieve this gold standard, where high dosages of isotope are delivered to the tumour. The steps that have been taken to try to achieve this ideal are described in this chapter.

STATE OF THE ART—LIMITATIONS OF RADIOLABELLED MONOCLONAL ANTIBODIES

A large number of experimental studies, based on the nude mouse and human cancer xenograft have been carried out. These have demonstrated the specificity of radiolabelled antibodies to localise to tumours and defined the absolute amount of radiolabel taken up per unit of tumour tissue. In some examples, up to 25% of the radioiodine labelled monoclonal antibody has been detected per gram of tumour with only minimal uptake by normal mouse organs [3]. These early results were very encouraging and as a result following higher dosages of iodine-131 antibodies, tumour regression was seen in experimental models [5].

Unfortunately, only a limited number of clinical studies have been carried out, which have examined the biological distribution and absolute amount of radiolabelled antibody uptake by tumour and normal organs in patients with cancer. We undertook such an investigation using three different tumour associated monoclonal antibodies (HMFG2, AUA1 and H17E2) and showed that the amounts of radioiodine labelled tumour associated monoclonal antibodies reaching their target tissues, after intravenous administration, were small [6]. It was of interest that lymph node metastases showed higher uptake than primary tumours [7]. The amounts of isotope targeted using radioiodine labelled antibodies were too small to be exploited therapeutically. That finding was disappointing, in view of the expectation that monoclonal antibodies should have performed better than traditional polyclonal antisera. Nevertheless, the ratio of uptake of label in tumour as compared to normal tissue was sufficiently high to be potentially useful for specific imaging of neoplastic lesions, using conventional gamma camera scanning [7] (Figs 6.1 and 6.2).

There are a number of reasons for this comparative failure to localise to human target tissues. The relative amounts of injected

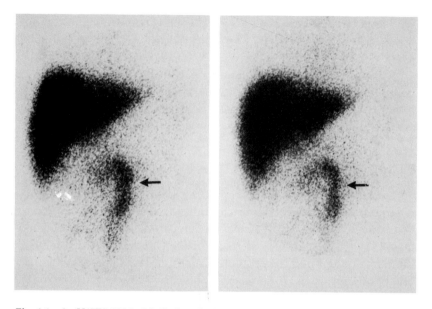

Fig. 6.1   An H17E2-111-In-labelled antibody scan taken (a) at 24 hours and (b) 48 hours after injection in a patient with testicular tumour metastatic to the paraaortic lymph nodes (arrows).

antibodies are much higher in animals than in humans and it is possible that the low tumour uptake in patients may be due to a dilution factor. If this is true, then one would need to use greater amounts of monoclonal antibodies than currently applied, amounts in the region of 20–25 mg of immunoglobulin per patient. This is now possible because of the development of large scale tissue culture techniques and advances in the production of high yields of immunoglobulin from small volume of supernatant.

A further explanation for the low amounts of monoclonal antibodies targeted to tumour may be because, although in experimental models, monoclonal antibodies tend to be truly tumour specific, in patients it is possible that there is cross reactivity with normal tissues. No tumour specific antigens have been found and it is not expected that tumours, with the exception of B cell lymphoma, bear unique markers. It may be that monoclonal antibodies are catabolised before they localise to tumours. Although mouse immunoglobulin catabolism by humans has not been thoroughly studied, it is probable that most of this is carried out, by the reticulo-endothelial system. It is possible that the catabolism of the radiolabel may vary considerably from

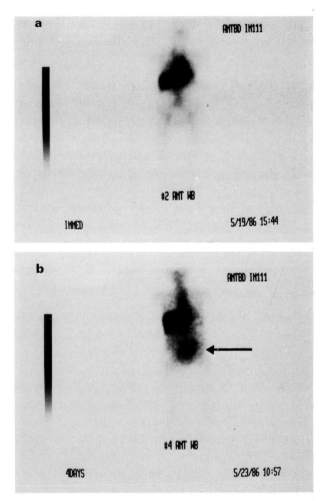

Fig. 6.2 An OVTL3-111-In-labelled antibody scan taken (a) immediately and (b) at 4 days after injection in a patient with ovarian cancer (arrow).

isotope to isotope. Therefore, important considerations for improved antibody guided tumour imaging and therapy include, choice of antigen and epitope, choice of antibody, choice of radiolabel, choice of radiolabelling method, possible pre-treatment of the host for the purpose of antigenic modulation, or specific immunosuppression, and finally choice of route of antibody administration. Ultimately, one could consider a structured approach of radiolabelled antibody treatment combined with other therapeutic modalities such as surgery, chemotherapy, external beam irradiation, hormones or biological response modifying agents.

TUMOUR ANTIGENS

In the current situation where tumour specific antigens have not been defined in most malignancies, it is still possible to produce monoclonal antibodies against various epitopes on tumour associated antigens. These antigens may be found on some normal tissues, but their differential expression on tumours is greater, allowing their use as tumour markers.

In the following section we will refer to specific molecules that play an essential role in some neoplasms. These offer a source for investigation and research and enable us to understand the processes of neoplastic transformation.

Placental alkaline phosphatase

Alkaline phosphatases are glycoproteins that catalyse the hydrolysis of monophosphate esters at high pH. They are bound on cell membranes and occur in various forms in different tissues. In humans there are three isoenzymic forms, the placental, the intestinal and the liver/bone/kidney, initially named for the organ in which they were first identified. At least three gene loci appear to encode the protein moieties of the three different alkaline phosphatases [8].

Placental alkaline phosphatase (orthophosphoric-monoester phosphohydrolase (alkaline optimum), E.C. 3.1.3.1-PLAP) can be distinguished from the two other major forms of AP by its unusual heat stability, differential inhibition, immunological reactivity and electrophoretic pattern.

PLAP is a cell-surface associated enzyme [9]. It is a relatively late evolutionary gene product normally synthesised by syncytio-trophoblasts from the twelfth week of pregnancy under control of the foetal genotype [10]. PLAP is composed of two subunits each with molecular weight of approximately 65 000 and can be liberated from cells by proteolytic cleavage by bromelain or trypsin. Bromelain results in the loss of a 2000 (10 000 for trypsin) molecular weight peptide from the PLAP subunit, which is thought to be the membrane binding component of PLAP. This bromelain-mediated cleavage is specific for the placental and intestinal form of alkaline phosphatase, while the liver/bone/kidney form is resistant [11].

A great deal of the interest in PLAP stems from the observation by Fishmann [12] and Nakayama [13], that isoenzymic forms of PLAP are ectopically expressed in cancer cells. The ectopic appearance of PLAP and PLAP-like isoenzymes is a useful marker of differentiation in human testicular cancer. Very high amounts of PLAP have been described in seminomas and certain other testicular tumours [14], as well as in prostate and bladder carcinomas [15, 16]. The presence of this enzyme has been also described in epidermoid carcinomas [17], adenocarcinomas [18], choriocarcinomas [15], lung [19], breast, pancreas, cervix [15] and colon carcinomas [15]. High serum levels of PLAP have also been found in patients with seminoma [20]. Alkaline phosphatases with enzymatic and immunologic properties similar to PLAP have been identified in small amounts in normal testicular tissue, cervix, lung, thymus and female genital organs [21, 22]. It is not yet clear if the gene expressed in malignant cells is the same as the one encoding normal PLAP. The recent availability of PLAP cDNA and knowledge of its chromosomal location should allow further studies of this gene family and its relationship with human disease [23]. Clinically placental alkaline phosphatase appears to be an excellent target for diagnostic and therapeutic purposes.

Human milk fat globule membrane

The human milk fat globules (HMFG) are surrounded by membranes which are representative of the differentiation stage of the secretory mammary cell. The cream fraction of human milk provides a ready source of this membrane which contains more than 15 components of which the most immunogenic is a large glycoprotein (300 000 in molecular weight) consisting of at least 50% carbohydrate [24]. The smaller molecular weight components that are also found are probably precursors of the larger glycoprotein. On the HMFG membrane another antigen is found which is the precursor of the blood group antigens [25].

Antisera to membrane preparations of HMFG have been used in the past to identify normal mammary epithelial cells in culture, and to demonstrate the presence of differentiation antigens on mammary cancers and normal lactating breast. Several monoclonal antibodies have been produced, and used in the diagnosis and treatment of malignant disease [26, 27]. It is of interest that apart from breast, other neoplastic tissues capable of secretory activity express such antigens.

Monoclonal antibodies directed to HMFG membrane antigens have a broad spectrum of cross reactivity with neoplasms of epithelial origin, particularly ovary, cervix, lung, uterus, thyroid and gastrointestinal tract [28, 29]. Such antigens are not tumour specific, because they are weakly expressed in resting breast, as well as on some other normal epithelial tissues with mainly secretory functions, such as sebaceous glands, salivary glands, exocrine pancreas, bile duct, cervix, ovary, endometrium and kidney [30].

Carcinoembryonic antigen

Carcinoembryonic antigen (CEA) is a foetal colon cell surface glycoprotein. It is normally present in foetal gut, liver and pancreas, and abnormally expressed in neoplastic adult tissues.

CEA was first defined by Gold and Freedman [31], as an antigen associated with neoplastic and embryonic gastrointestinal tissues, with a molecular weight of 180–200 000. It is now clear that CEA is not a single molecular component, but a heterogeneous group of glycoproteins [32]. CEA may not be tumour specific, but the fact that its concentration is high in a variety of epithelial malignancies such as colonic, gastric, cervical, ovarian and lung carcinomas allows its use as a target for tumour localisation [33].

There are limitations in the application of monoclonal antibodies directed to CEA. CEA is a heterogeneous molecule, and several anti-CEA antibodies have been produced that recognise different epitopes [34]. CEA is not uniformly distributed so that within the same tumour some cells are positive while others are negative. There is a cross reactivity with a normal tissue component termed non-specific cross reactive antigen (NCA) that has been extracted from normal adult tissues, meconium [35] and faeces [36]. Some anti-CEA monoclonal antibodies may cross react with normal liver or with granulocytes [36]. Finally, the fact that CEA is a shed antigen limits the use of anti-CEA monoclonal antibodies because of possible antibody-antigen complex formation in the circulation or in the microenvironment of the tumour. The above mentioned problems however are relevant to most tumour associated antigens, and are not unique to CEA.

THE CHOICE OF ANTIBODY

The technique currently used for raising monoclonal antibodies is basically the same as that originally described by Kohler and Milstein in 1975 [37]. Mice or rats are immunised with the appropriate antigen, and their spleen cells are then fused with myeloma cells in the presence of polyethylene glycol.

The choice of animal to be immunised will be determined by the source of the antigen. The immunised animal must be from another species and the immunogen must be an alloantigen in order to be easily recognised as foreign. The selection of the animal host will also be affected by the choice of myeloma cell line, since intra-species hybrids are more stable than inter-species one.

Rodents therefore are widely in use, and among them, mice and rats are the most popular. Most monoclonal antibodies are of mouse origin and this is because the mouse system was the first to be developed. Mice or rats are easy to handle, and it has been shown that they recognise certain epitopes expressed on human malignancies. Moreover, a wide range of myeloma cell lines are now available; the most frequently used are the mouse Ag8 (P3×63-AG8−653) and NS-1 (53/NS-1/1-Ag4-1) and the rat Y3 (Y3-AG1.2.3) and YO (YB2/3.0Ag20). The most suitable ones are the mouse Ag8 and rat Y3 because of their inability to synthesise their own immunoglobulin-heavy and light chains.

In addition to the development of rodent monoclonal antibodies human monoclonal antibodies have also been developed [8]. Human immune responses to mouse antibodies can interfere with subsequent murine antibody administration, and lead to allergic reactions [39]. Human monoclonal antibodies may reduce this problem [40]. One cannot immunise humans with cancer cells for fear of cancer transmission, but there are several alternative approaches to the production of human monoclonal antibodies. One strategy that has been attempted is the fusion of human lymphocytes, with myeloma cells. The lymphocytes that were used were the ones present in the tumour or around it and the myelomas were the traditional NS-1, Ag8 or Y3 lines [41]. Human myeloma lines were not used because of the difficulty in growing them in culture. A number of human monoclonal antibodies have been produced with good specificity especially to mammary [42] lung, prostate and cervix cancers [43, 44] as well as to gliomas [45].

Another approach to human monoclonal antibody production is the transfection and immortalisation of suitable human lymphocytes with Epstein–Barr Virus (EBV) *in vitro*, so that the lymphocytes will continuously secrete immunoglobulin [46]. Suitable lymphocytes are isolated by rosetting with antigen-coupled erythrocytes; or in the presence of antigen-coupled to fluorescein, by fluorescence-activated cell sorter; or by secondary *in vitro* stimulation with antigen.

Unfortunately technical problems have made the production of human monoclonal antibodies difficult. The combined techniques of EBV transformed lymphocytes and conventional fusion, or immortalisation by gene transfer, has been attempted. However, it is too early to know if the production of human monoclonal antibodies will provide advances in hybridoma technology.

Passive immunotherapy with monoclonal antibodies maybe effective in the treatment of solid tumours. On the other hand radiolabelled monoclonal antibodies may be more effective, because radioactivity can kill nearby cells that have not been targetted by antibody. There is no need to use monoclonal antibodies of a specific subclass, or even the whole IgG molecule, which will elicit a more marked anti-mouse response [39]. Fragmentation has been used to remove the Fc portion from the Ab molecule. Pepsin can cleave off the Fc region, leaving the two Fab fragments bound together in a bivalent structure [F(ab')$_2$]. Papain on the other hand removes a large portion of the heavy chains, the constant region, leaving two monovalent Fab fragments [47]. Fab fragments being monovalent are of a lower avidity than F(ab')$_2$ and hence the latter are more commonly in use. F(ab')$_2$ fragments have less non-specific uptake than the whole IgG and a shorter half life in the blood, both of which favour the use of fragments as compared with the whole Ig molecule.

The production of heterobispecific antibodies (hybrid monoclonal antibodies) may offer potential advantages. Hybrid antibodies are IgGs, that have two different hypervariable regions, directed either against two different epitopes of the same antigen, or two completely different antigens. Avidity and tumour uptake may be increased and normal tissues decreased by the use of this type of antibody.

Production of hybrid antibodies can be achieved chemically, by reducing under mild conditions the disulphide bonds of the IgGs and then reassociating two different half molecules through that bond or by using hybridoma techniques and fusing two different clones. The new hybridomas may possess the specificities of each parent molecule [48].

THE CHOICE OF RADIOISOTOPE

Radionuclides used for imaging with radiolabelled antibodies should ideally be characterised by a physical half life of 6 hours to 8 days; gamma energy range of 20–240 Kev; high single energy gamma abundance per decay; small abundances and low energy particulate radiation; good radiolabelling properties; and stability. Radiolabelled antibodies selected as therapeutic agents should have complementary properties. However, their decay should be mainly via particulate radiation with little or no accompanying gamma radiation.

Monoclonal antibodies can be labelled with radionuclides using established radioiodination techniques [49] or by newer conjugation methods [50]. Iodine-125 is most often used to determine relative tissue distribution in pre-clinical studies. Scintillation camera imaging can be performed with Iodine-125 in small animals, but Iodine-123 is more appropriate for clinical studies. The 13 hours half life of Iodine-123 restricts its use to short-term studies, but excellent images can be obtained from its favourable gamma emmission. Iodine-131 unfortunately, is of limited clinical potential, despite its low cost and ready availability. Effective radiolabels, other than iodine, have been developed but their half lives and residence times must be carefully matched with the needs of both imaging and therapy. Indium-111 and Technetium-99m are examples of radionuclides that are currently under extensive investigation. Bromine-77, Cobalt-55 and Copper-67 are potentially interesting cyclotron produced radionuclides.

Copper-69, Yttrium-90, Rhenium-186 and Astatine-211 have possible therapeutic application since strong particle radiations are associated with their decay. Yttrium-90 and Rhenium-186 are thought to be among the best radiolabels for therapy as they possess a sufficiently long half life for tumour localisation, little or no gamma radiation, stable daughter products, and can form stable chelates with antibodies [51].

Palladium-109, a beta emitting radionuclide, was chelated by Fawwaz et al. [52] to a monoclonal antibody against the high molecular weight melanoma associated antigen. Injection of the radiolabelled monoclonal antibody into nude mice bearing human melanoma resulted in significant accumulation of the radiolabel in the tumour. These authors suggested that this Palladium-109 labelled monoclonal might have a potential application in tumour therapy. Scandium-47 may also be useful for radioimmunotherapy and imaging [53]. Bismuth-212 has been proposed as a therapeutic radiolabel due to the extremely high linear energy transfer of its alpha emissions and its availability as a generator product of Lead-212. The 1 hour half life of Bismuth-212 limits its application but Lead-212, with its 11 hours' half life, may be a more appropriate antibody label. Copper-67 with its 62 hour half life, is already under investigation as a therapeutic agent [54]. Phosphorous-32 should be theoretically superior to Iodine-131 for treatment because it is a pure beta emitter; has a higher energy; and has a long physical half life [55]. Gallium-67 offers little advantage over Indium-111 for single photon imaging, but Gallium-68 may be useful for studies with positron emission tomography. Various stable elements such as manganese and gadolinium have been studied in nuclear magnetic resonance imaging (MRI) [56].

Boron neutron capture therapy (BNCT) combines the attractive features of both external beam and internal radioisotope therapy to deliver a large differential dose to boron-loaded tumour cells interspersed within healthy tissue [57]. Despite the failure of early trials there may be a place for monoclonal antibodies in the treatment of tumours with BNCT if a method can be developed that can allow for a high number of boron molecules (>100) to be attached onto a molecule of antibody.

From the existing data, radiolabelled monoclonal antibodies can only be advocated as a radiation therapy 'boost' or for the treatment of micrometastases. By this method, it may be possible to deliver 1000–1500 cGy to a tumour. However, until improved targeting with at least a ten-fold improvement in antibody uptake is achieved, the potentially widespread and effective use of therapeutic radioactive antibodies cannot be realised.

RADIOLABELLING METHODS

The chosen method of conjugation must allow controlled incorporation and optimal preservation of radionuclide and antibody activities. Coupling reactions specific for amino acid residues may lead to the antigen binding site being blocked and loss of immunoreactivity. Two moieties in immunoglobulins may provide linkage sites not likely to interfere with the binding site. One is the carbohydrate group usually present in the constant regions of heavy chains and only occasionally in the variable region. The other linkage site can be provided by free sulphhydryl groups formed following reductive cleavage of the interchain disulphide bridges in immunoglobulins.

Monoclonal antibodies can be labelled with iodine using several electron acceptors. Chloramine-T [58] and iodogen [59] have been two of the most commonly used methods. Newer radioiodination techniques using the mild oxidant N-bromosuccinimide [60] or the Bolton–Hunter reagent [61] may have further advantages.

The actual number of iodine atoms that can be attached per molecule of antibody is dependent on the number of tyrosine moieties available for iodination. Proteins like antibodies may be altered by radiolabelling, therefore special care must be taken in the preparation of labelled antibodies so as not to lose immunoreactivity.

The attachment of metal ions to monoclonal antibodies by means of bifunctional agents appears to be of potential in the preparation of new cancer imaging and therapeutic agents. Diethylenetriamine pentaacetic acid (DTPA), is a bifunctional reagent that is most commonly used [62]. It chelates with metallic cations such as Indium-111 and Yttrium-90 and it is easy to use because there is no need for intermediates. There are many forms of DTPA such as the cyclic dianhydrate, the carboxycarbonic anhydride, the o-acylisourea, the N-hydroxysuccinamide penta ester (DHSE), or the N-hydroxysuccinamide active ester. By increasing the DTPA per antibody molar ratio, one can get better labelling results, but this may lead to dimer or polymer formation, resulting in higher non-specific liver uptake and human anti-monoclonal antibody response. Ethylenediaminotetraacetic acid (EDTA) has also been used as Benzyl-EDTA, or bromoacetamidobenzyl EDTA (BABE) (63), without significant differences from DTPA.

Unfortunately the problem of transchelation *in vivo* to transferrin and other proteins still remains, and this leads to the 9% per day overall loss for Indium-111 and 13% for Yttrium-90. Moreover the kinetic liability of certain metal ions, poses special problems [63]. New macrocyclic bifunctional metal chelators have therefore been synthesised, such as p-nitro-benzyl TETA or its derivative p-bromoacetamido-benzyl TETA (TETA = 1,4,8,11 tetraazacyclotetradecane-NN^1 N^{11}N^{111} tetraacetic acid) [64]. Such macrocyclic structures bind to metals making them more stable *in vivo* than chelates of EDTA or DTPA [64]. Conjugates can also be made using intermediaries, such as polyglutamine acid, polylysine, various polysaccharides and synthetic polymers. Polytyrosines can potentially be linked to antibodies allowing higher specific activities.

ROUTES OF ANTIBODY ADMINISTRATION

The problems associated with successful radioimmunotherapy are for the most part an extension of those facing antibody guided imaging. The use of intra-arterial, intracavitary, subcutaneous and intra-lymphatic routes of administration can direct antibodies to regionally confined tumours. If an antibody is administered into a restricted space such as the pleural, pericardial or peritoneal cavity [65], it should be possible to achieve higher uptake by the tumour target, lower uptake by normal organs, and reduced uptake in the liver and the reticulo-endothelial system which are involved in immunoglobulin catabolism. Injection of radioactive materials into serous cavities has been attempted previously [66] but proved only partly effective firstly because of the inability of the radioactive material to reach all the cancer cells and secondly because of its 'normal removal' by macro-phages and other leukocytes. The specificity and intrinsic affinity of tumour associated monoclonal antibodies should make them superior to non-specific agents such as radioactive colloids which are conven-tionally used to deliver radiation.

Antibody guided irradiation of malignant lesions has been at-tempted in the past with only limited success. We have recently re-ported that the regional rather than the systemic infusion of radioac-tively labelled tumour associated monoclonal antibodies can produce favourable results in the treatment of some malignant diseases such as ovarian cancer [67]. Intracavitary administration of radiolabelled tumour associated monoclonal antibodies has been used in an attempt to avoid 'first pass' catabolism of antibodies by blood and the reticulo-endothelial system. Intraperitoneal delivery of monoclonal antibodies offers considerable advantage over intravenous administration, espe-cially in the early hours after injection [67].

Monoclonal antibody guided irradiation delivered by arterial in-fusion to the tumour area may be of clinical value in the treatment of brain gliomas and some other tumours, resistant to conventional forms of treatment. Cases reported from Hammersmith Hospital [68] showed that radiolabelled tumour associated monoclonal antibody given by an internal carotid arterial infusion can result in tumour regression and may be of value in relieving the symptoms and improving the quality of life in recurrent high grade glioma resistant to conventional forms of treatment. Further studies are now needed to examine the reproducibility of these reports and estimate the long term benefit, if any, to patients with brain tumours resistant to conventional treatment.

When the objective is to detect or to treat tumour in regional lymph nodes, intralymphatic injection may be effective. Monoclonal antibodies enter local lymphatic capillaries, pass to the draining lymph nodes, and may bind to target cells. Antibody not bound in the first node group encountered passes to more distant nodes. If not removed from the lymph node, the antibody passes into the blood stream. Weinstein et al. [67] suggested that when the aim is to diagnose or treat early lymph node metastases, the lymphatic route provides higher sensitivity, lower background, lower systemic toxicity and faster localisation than the intravenous route. More interestingly the lymphatic route minimises exposure of antibody to cross reactive antigen present on normal tissues elsewhere in the body so that lower doses may be used for diagnosis or therapy. This may decrease the systemic toxicity of antibodies and allow the imaging of smaller masses, with reduced body background. Because of the direct entry of antibody into the lymphatics, nodal images may appear within minutes after injection without the need to await clearance from the blood stream [69]. The most serious limitation of lymphatic delivery is the regional nature of the approach and the restriction to lymph nodes that drain the site of injection [70].

CONCLUSIONS AND FUTURE PROSPECTS

We require more effective, less toxic and highly specific cancer treatments and this may be provided by tumour specific monoclonal antibodies. This is because the extraordinary resolving power of monoclonal antibodies permits the detailed dissection of antigens and epitopes on cancer cells. Monoclonal antibodies can be produced in great quantities and this allows their clinical application. The potential role of monoclonal antibodies in the management of cancer is broad based and includes diagnosis, prognosis and therapy. It may be that the use of a cocktail of monoclonal antibodies in combination may be of advantage, compared to single antibody preparations [71]. Greater knowledge of the structure and function of antigens and the development of new methods of altering antigen expression [72] will aid the selection of appropriate agents for diagnosis and treatment.

Three major problems limit the use of monoclonal antibodies in tumour therapy. These are the antigenic heterogeneity of neoplasms, the small amount of antibody targeted in tumours and the development of a human anti-murine immune immunoglobulin response. The problem of heterogeneity may be dealt with either by the use of cocktails of monoclonal antibodies or by altering differentiation states. Energetic beta emitting radioisotopes could be applied to destroy a 'tumour area' rather than a single tumour cell and the use of these agents could avoid the problems of limited tumour antibody targeting. One approach to reduce the problem of a human anti-murine globulin response is to use antibody fragments instead of intact IgG [73]. Another approach is to use human monoclonal antibodies, but these are difficult to prepare [74]. It is now possible by using recombinant DNA techniques to obtain antibodies where the antigen binding site is defined by sequences from a rodent monoclonal antibody but the rest of the molecule is of human origin. Boulianne and Morrison [75] were the first to describe the production of functional chimaeric antibodies and since then several others have been able to achieve this using a variety of tumour associated rodent monoclonal antibodies. This approach can be extended much further; Neuberger [76] showed that the Fc portion of the antibody can be replaced by other unrelated proteins such as an enzyme thus developing new molecules with novel effector functions.

In this chapter we have outlined the progress achieved so far, using monoclonal antibodies. Nevertheless, many difficulties remain especially in identifying appropriate antigens, developing optimal antibody species, attaching the most effective radiolabel or cytotoxic agent to antibody and choosing the best method of administration.

REFERENCES

1 Hericourt, J. and Richet, C. Traitement d'un cas de sarcome par la serotherapie. C R Hebal Seances Acad Sci. 1895, **120**: 948–950.

2 Pressman, D. and Keighley, G. The zone of activity of antibodies as determined by the use of radioactive tracers; the zone of activity of nephrotoxic anti-kidney serum. J Immunol. 1948, **59**: 141–146.

3 Ballou, B., Levine, G., Hakala, R.J. and Solker D. Tumour localisation detected with radioactively labelled monoclonal antibody and external scintigraphy. Science. 1979, **206**: 844–846.

4 Mach, J.P., Buchegger, F., Forni, M. et al. Use of ^{131}I radiolabelled monoclonal anti-CEA antibodies for the detection of human carcinomas by external photo-scanning and tomoscintigraphy. Immunol Today. 1981, **2**: 239–249.

5 Farrands, P.A., Perkins, A.C., Pimm, M.V. et al. Radioimmunodetection of human colorectal cancer by an antitumour monoclonal antibody. Lancet. 1982, **ii**: 397–400.

6 Epenetos, A.A., Courtenay-Luck, N., Halnan, K.E. *et al.* Antibody guided irradiation of malignant lesions. *Lancet.* 1984, **30**: 1441–1443.

7 Wilson, C.B. and Epenetos, A.A. Use of monoclonal antibodies for diagnosis and treatment of liver tumours. *Baillière's Clin Gastroenterol.* 1987, **1**: 115–130.

8 Seargeant, L.E. and Stinson, R.A. Evidence that three structural genes code for human alkaline phosphatases. *Nature.* 1979, **281**: 152–154.

9 Tokumitsu, S., Tokumitsu, K., Kohnoe, K. *et al.* Localisation of alkaline phosphatase isoenzymes in human cancer cells *in vitro. Acta Histochem Cytochem.* 1979, **12**: 631.

10 Fishmann, L., Miyayanua, H., Driscoll, S.G. *et al.* Developmental phase-specific alkaline-phosphatase isoenzymes of human placenta and their occurrence in human cancer. *Cancer Res.* 1976, **36**: 2268–2273.

11 Hanford, W.C. and Fishmann, W.H. Measurement of biosynthetic and intracellular transit times for a cell-surface membrane glycoprotein, alkaline phosphatase in Hela cells. *Anal Biochem.* 1983, **129**: 176–183.

12 Fishmann, W.H., Inglis, N.R., Stolbauch, L.L. *et al.* A serum alkaline phosphatase isoenzyme of human neoplastic cell origin. *Cancer Res.* 1968, **28**: 150–154.

13 Nakayama, T., Yoshidu, M. and Kitamura, M. L-leucine sensitive, heat stable alkaline-phosphatase isoenzyme detected in a patient with pleuritis carcinomatosa. *Clin Chim Acta.* 1970, **30**: 546–548.

14 Benham, F.J., Andrews, P.W., Knowles, B.B. *et al.* Alkaline phosphatase isoenzymes as possible markers of differentiation in human testicular teratocarcinoma cell lines. *Dev Biol.* 1981, **88**: 279–287.

15 Benham, F.J., Fogh, J. and Haris, H. Alkaline phosphatase expression on human cell lines derived from various malignancies. *Int J Cancer.* 1981, **27**: 637–644.

16 Herz, F. and Fox, L.G. Alkaline phosphatase activity in cultured urinary bladder cancer cells. *Arch Biochem Biophys.* 1979, **194**: 30–35.

17 Jemmerson, R., Shah, N., Takeya, M. *et al.* Characterisation of the placental alkaline phospatase-like (Nagao) isonenzyme on the surface of AU31 human epidermoid carcinoma cells. *Cancer Res.* 1985, **45**: 282–287.

18 Jemmerson, R., Shah, N. and Fishmann, W.H. Evidence for homology of normal and neoplastic human placental alkaline phosphatases as determined by monoclonal antibodies to the cancer associated enzyme. *Cancer Res.* 1985, **45**: 3268–3273.

19 Loose, J.H., Damjanov, I. and Harris, H. Identity of the neoplastic alkaline phospatase as revealed with monoclonal antibodies to the placental form of the enzyme. *Am J Clin Pathol.* 1984, **82(2)**: 173–177.

20 Jeppson, A., Wahren, B., Brehmer-Anderson, E., *et al.* Eutopic expression of placental alkaline phosphatase in testicular tumours. *Int J Cancer.* 1984, **34**: 757–761.

21 Goldstein, D.J., Rogers, C. and Harris, H. A search for trace expression of placental-like alkaline phosphatase in non-malignant human tissues: demonstration of its occurrence in lung, cervix, testis and thymus. *Clin Chim Acta.* 1982, **125**: 63–75.

22 Nozawa, S., Ohta, H., Izumi, S. *et al.* Heat stable alkaline phosphatase in the

normal female genital organ–with special reference to the histochemical heat-stability test and L-Phe inhibition test. *Acta Histochem Cytochem.* 1980, **13(5)**: 521–530.

23 Kam, W., Clauser, E., Kim, Y.S. *et al.* Cloning sequencing, and chromosomal localisation of human term placental alkaline phosphatase. *Proc Natl Acad Sci USA.* 1985, **82**: 8715–8719.

24 Shimizu, M. and Yamanchi, K. Isolation and characterisation of mucin-like glycoprotein in human milk fat globule membrane. *J Biochem.* 1982, **91**: 515–524.

25 Gooi, H.C., Uemaura, K., Edwards, P.A.W. *et al.* Two mouse hybridoma antibodies against HMFG recognise the I (MA) antigenic determinant beta-D-Galpl–beta-D-GlcpNAc 1->6. *Carbohydr Res.* 1983, **120**: 293–302.

26 Taylor-Papadimitriou, J., Peterson, J.A., Arklie, J. *et al.* Monoclonal antibodies to epithelium-specific components of the HMGF membrane: production and reaction with cells in culture. *Int J Cancer.* 1981, **28**: 17–21.

27 Ceriani, R.L., Sasaki, M., Sussman, H. *et al.* Circulating human mammary epithelial antigens in breast cancer. *Proc Natl Acad Sci USA.* 1982, **79**: 5420–5424.

28 Epenetos, A.A., Shepherd, J., Britton, K.E. *et al.* I-123 radioiodinated antibody imaging of occult ovarian cancer. *Cancer.* 1985, **55(5)**: 984–987.

29 Epenetos, A.A. Antibody guided lymphangiography in the staging of cervical cancer. *Br J Cancer.* 1985, **51**: 805–808.

30 Taylor-Papadimitriou, J., and Griffiths, A.B. Development of monoclonal antibodies with specificity for human epithelial cells. In: Gregoriadis, A.G., Poste, G., Senior, J. and Trouet, A. (eds) *Receptor-mediated targetting of drugs.* New York Plenum Press, 1984, 201–234.

31 Gold, P. and Freedman, S.O. Specific carcinoembryonic antigens of the human digestive system. *J Exp Med.* 1965, **121**: 439–462.

32 Von Kleist, S. and Burtin, P. Antigens cross-reacting with CEA. In: Herberman, R.B. and McIntyre, C.K. (eds) *Immunodiagnosis of Cancer*, New York: Marcel Dekker Inc, 1979, 322–342.

33 Ford, C.H.J., Newman, C.E., Johnson, J.R. *et al.* Localisation and toxicity study of a Vindesin-anti CEA conjugate in patients with advanced cancer. *Br J Cancer*, 1983, **47**: 35–42.

34 Primus, F.J., Kuhr W.J. and Goldenberg, D.M. Immunological hetergeneity of CEA: immunohistochemical detection of CEA determinants in colonic tumours with mAbs. *Cancer Res.* 1983, **43**: 693–701.

35 Primus, F.J., Freeman, J.W. and Goldenberg, D.M. Immunological hetero-geneity of CEA: purification from meconium of antigen related to CEA. *Cancer Res.* 1983, **43**: 679–685.

36 Wagener, C., Young, Y.H.Z., Crawford, F.G. *et al.* Monoclonal antibodies for CEA and related antigens as a model system: a systematic approach for the determination of epitope specificities of monoclonal antibodies. *J Immunol.* 1983, **130**: 2308–2315.

37 Köhler, G. and Milstein, C. Continuous cultures of fused cells secreting anti-body of predefined specificity. *Nature.* 1975, **256**: 495–497.

38 Cote, R.J., Morissey, D.M., Houghton, A.N. *et al.* Generation of human mono-clonal antibodies reactive with cellular antigens. *Proc Natl Acad Sci USA.* 1983, **80**: 2026–2030.

39 Schroff, R.W., Foon, K.A., Shannon, B.M. *et al.* Human anti-murine immuno-globulin responses in patients receiving monoclonal antibody therapy. *Cancer Res.* 1985, **45**: 879–885.

40 Sikora, K. Human monoclonal antibodies. *Br Med Bull.* 1984, **40(3)**: 209–212.

41 Yasuda, K., Alderson, T., Phillips, J. *et al.* Detection of lymphocytes infiltrating gliomas by monoclonal antibodies. *J Neur Neurosurg Psychiatry.* 1983, **46**: 734–737.

42 Schlom, J., Wunderlich, D. and Teramoto, Y.A. Generation of monoclonal antibodies reactive with human mammary carcinomas. *Proc Natl Acad Sci USA.* 1980, **77**: 6841–6845.

43 Glassy, M.C., Handley, H.H., Hagiwara, H. *et al.* UC-729-6-a human lympho-blastoid line useful for generating antibody secreting human-human hybrid-omas. *Proc Natl Acad Sci USA.* 1983, **80**: 6327–6331.

44 Hagiwane, H. and Sato, G.H. Human-human hybridoma producing mono-clonal antibody against autologous cervical carcinoma. *Mol Biol Med.* 1983, **1(2)**: 245–252.

45 Sikora, K., Alderson, T., Phillips, T. *et al.* Human hybridomas to malignant gliomas. *Lancet.* 1982, **1**: 11–14.

46 Kozbor, D. and Roder, J.C. Requirements for the establishment of high filtered human monoclonal antibodies against tetanus toxoid using the EBV technique. *J Immunol.* 1981, **127**: 1275–1280.

47 Moldofsky, P.S., Powe, J., Mulhern, C.B. *et al.* Metastatic colon carcinoma detected with radiolabelled F(ab')$_2$ monoclonal antibody fragments. *Radiol.* 1983, **149**: 549–555.

48 Galfre, G., Milstein, C. and Wright, B. Rat x rat hybrid myelomas and a monoclonal anti-Fd portion of mouse IgG. *Nature.* 1979, **277**: 131–133.

49 Keenaiι, A.M. *et al.* Monoclonal antibodies in nuclear medicine. *J Nucl Med.* 1985, **26(5)**: 531–537.

50 Childs, R.L. and Hnatowich, D.J. Optimum conditions for labelling of DTPA-coupled antibodies with technitium-99m. *J Nucl Med.* 1985, **26(3)**: 293–299.

51 Beirwalters, W.H. Horizons in radionuclide therapy: 1985 update. *J Nucl Med.* 1985, **26**: 421–427.

52 Fawwaz, R.E. *et al.* Potential of Palladium-109-labelled antimelanoma mono-clonal antibody for tumour therapy. *J Nucl Med.* 1984, **25**: 796–799.

53 Anderson, W.T. and Strand, M. Stability targeting and biodistribution of scan-dium-46 and gallium-67-labelled monoclonal antibody to erythroleukemic mice. *Cancer Res.* 1985, **45**: 2154–2158.

54 Cole, W. *et al.* Development of Copper-67 chelate conjugated monoclonal anti-bodies for radioimmunotherapy. *J Nucl Med.* 1983, **24**: p30 (Abstr).

55 Foxwell, B.M.J. Antibody-kemptide conjugate: A novel method for the 32P-labelling of monoclonal antibodies. *Br J Cancer.* 1986, **54**: 536 (Abstr).

56 Courtet, C., Bourgoin, C., Bohy, J. *et al.* MR1 after injection of specific NMR contrast agent Gd-25 DTPA—MAb in nude mice bearing human colon adenocarcinoma. *Br J Cancer.* 1987, **56**: 5240 (Abstr).

57 Fairchild, R.G., Elmore, J.J., Borg, D.C. *et al.* Bolon-10-labelled antibodies for neutron capture therapy. *Br J Cancer.* 1984, **50**: 562–564.

58 Hunter, W.M. and Greenwood, F.C. Preparation of iodine-131 labelled human growth hormone of high specific activity. *Nature.* 1962, **194**: 495–496.

59 Fraker, P.J. and Speck, J.C. Jr. Proteins and cell membrane iodinations with a sparingly soluble chloroglycoluril. *Biochem Biophys Res Comm.* 1978, **80**: 849–857.

60 Reay, P. Use of N-bromosuccinimide for the iodination of proteins for radioimmunoassay. *Ann Clin Biochem.* 1982, **19**: 129–133.

61 Bolton, A.E. and Hunter, W.M. The labelling of proteins to high specific radioactivities by conjugation to a ^{125}I containing acylating agent. *Biochem J.* 1973, **133**: 529–539.

62 Krejcarek, G.E. and Tucker, K.L. Covalent attachement of chelating groups to macromolecules. *Biochem Biophys Res Comm.* 1977, **77**: 581–585.

63 Gobuty, A.H., Kim, E.E. and Weiner, R.E. Radiolabelled monoclonal antibodies: radiochemical pharmacokinetic and clinical challenges. *J Nucl Med.* 1985, **26(5)**: 546–548.

64 Moi, H.K., Meares, C.F., McCall, M.J. *et al.* Copper chelates as probes of biological systems: stable copper complexes with a macrocyclic bifuncional chelating agent. *Anal Biochem.* 1985, **148**: 249–253.

65 Epenetos, A.A., Munro, A.S., Stewart, S. *et al.* Antibody guided irradiation of advanced ovarian cancer with intraperitoneally administered radiolabelled monoclonal antibodies. *J Clin Oncol.* 1987, **5**: 1890–1899.

66 Muller, J.M. Uber die Verwendung von kunstlichen radioktiven Isotopen zur Erzielung von lokalisierten biologischen strahlen Wirkungen. *Experienta.* 1945, **6**: 199–200.

67 Weinstein, J.N. *et al.* Monoclonal antitumour antibodies in the lymphatics. *Cancer Treat Rep.* 1984, **68(1)**: 257–264.

68 Epenetos, A.A., Courtenay-Luck, N. and Pickering, D. *et al.* Antibody guided irradiation of brain glioma by arterial infusion of radioactive monoclonal antibody against epidermal growth factor receptor and blood group A antigen. *Br Med J.* 1985, **290**: 1463–1466.

69 Epenetos, A.A., Nimmon, C. and Arcklie, J. *et al.* Detection of human cancer in an animal model using radiolabelled tumour associated monoclonal antibodies. *Br J Cancer.* 1982, **46**: 1–5.

70 Taylor-Papadimitriou, J. *et al.* Monoclonal antibodies to epithelium-specific components of the human milk fat globule membrane: production and reaction with cells in culture. *Int J Cancer.* 1981, **28**: 17–21.

71 Munz, D.L., Alav, A., Koprowski, H. and Herlyn, D. Improved radioimaging of human tumour xenografts by a mixture of monoclonal antibody $F(ab')_2$ fragments. *J Nucl Med.* 1986, **27**: 1739–1745.

72 Rowlinson, G., Balkwill, F. and Snook, D. *et al.* Enhancement by gamma-interferon of *in-vivo* tumour localisation by a monoclonal antibody against HLA-DR antigen. *Cancer Res.* 1986, **46**: 6413–6417.

73 Buraggi, G.L., Callegaro, L. and Mariani, G. *et al.* Imaging with 131-I-labelled monoclonal antibodies to a high molecular weight melanoma associated antigen in patients with melanoma: efficacy of whole immunoglobulin and its $F(ab')_2$ fragments. *Cancer Res.* 1985, **46**: 3378–3387.

74 Sikora, K. Human monoclonal antibodies to cancer cells In: Strelkauskas, A.J. *Human Monoconal Antibodies.* New York: Marcel Dekker, 1985.

75 Boulianne, G.L., Hozumi, N. and Shulman, M.J. Production of functional chimaeric mouse/human antibodies. *Nature.* 1984, **312**: 643–646.

76 Neuberger, M.S., Williams, G.T. and Fox, R.O. Recombinant antibodies possessing novel effector functions. *Nature.* 1984, **312**: 604–612.

7 VIRUSES AND CERVICAL NEOPLASIA

J. TIDY AND P.J. FARRELL

OUR UNDERSTANDING of the role of viruses as aetiological agents in human cancer has rapidly increased over recent years. Epstein–Barr virus has been implicated in Burkitt's lymphoma [1] and nasopharyngeal carcinoma [2], hepatitis B in primary hepatocellular carcinoma [3], the human immunodeficiency virus HIV1 is associated with adult T cell leukaemias in Southern Japan [4], and skin cancers in patients with epidermodysplasia verruciformis are associated with human papilloma virus (HPV) types 5 and 8 [5, 6]. Infective agents have also been implicated in carcinoma of the cervix and these include *Treponema, Neisseria gonorrhoeae, Trichomonas,* chlamydia, cytomegalovirus, herpes simplex type 2 virus (HSV2) and human papillomavirus (HPV) [7, 8]. In 1983, Durst *et al.* [9] discovered that HPV16 was present in carcinoma of the cervix and this was the first clear link between papillomaviruses and a common human carcinoma that causes the death of 2000 women annually in England and Wales.

The first associations between infective agents and gynaecological cancer were described in the 19th century by Parent-Duchatelet who noted that there was a high incidence of syphilis, scabies and cancer of the uterus amongst prostitutes [10]. Recently Kessler, in controlled studies, found that there was a 2.7-fold increased risk of cervical neoplasia in women whose husbands had previously been married to a woman with cervical neoplasia [11]. As might be expected for a sexually transmitted disease, there is also an enhanced risk of development of cervical cancer in women whose husbands have multiple sexual partners [12, 13]. An increased rate of cervical cancer is also observed in the wives of men who have penile cancer [14, 15] and in the consorts of men with penile condylomas accumina have a higher incidence of cervical intraepithelial neoplasia (CIN) than age matched controls [16]. In this chapter we describe the significance of viral agents in cervical cancer.

HERPES SIMPLEX TYPE 2 VIRUS AND CARCINOMA OF THE CERVIX

Herpes simplex type 2 (HSV2) antigens and HSV associated RNAs have been detected occasionally in tumour specimens [17, 18] but HSV2 DNA has not consistently been found in the tumour genome. Biopsies from women with cervical neoplasia have been examined for both HSV2 and HPV DNAs. Fifteen per cent of invasive carcinomas were positive for HSV2 but no CIN was positive, while HPV DNA was detected in 65% of invasive carcinomas and 50% of CIN [19]. Recently McNab et al. [20] found HSV2 DNA to be present in the tumour genome in only one of 22 cases of carcinoma of the cervix. This low incidence of HSV2 has been explained by the 'hit and run' hypothesis which suggests that virus might transiently be present in the cell but is lost by the time the tumour clinically presents [21].

Several early seroepidemiological studies [22, 23] demonstrated that women with carcinoma of the cervix were more likely to have detectable antibodies to HSV2 than case controls. Vonka et al. [24] studied 10 000 women in Prague relating HSV2 antibody status, with cervical neoplasia. Almost 250 women with cervical neoplasia were matched with normal controls and no difference was found in the incidence of HSV2 antibodies between the two groups. It is now generally thought that the presence of HSV2 antibodies probably reflects sexual behaviour and that HSV2 infection is not the direct cause of cervical cancer. However, its role as a promotor or co-factor in carcinogenesis cannot be excluded.

HUMAN PAPILLOMAVIRUS AND CARCINOMA OF THE CERVIX

Morphological changes in both Papanicolaou smears and histological sections similar to those associated with papillomavirus infection were reported by Meisels and Fortin, and Purola and Savia [25, 26]. Both found that koilocytes (cells with a nuclear halo and irregular nuclei, known to be associated with papillomavirus infection) were present in 70% of specimens containing CIN1 and 2. Papillomavirus particles have been found in koilocytes by electron microscopy and im-munocytochemical staining [27].

Zur Hausen first suggested that HPV might be associated with carcinoma of the cervix in 1976 but it was not until 1983 that Durst *et al.* [9] demonstrated HPV16 in cervical tumours. Using DNA–DNA hybridisation techniques the virus was found in 61% of tumours examined from women in West Germany.

Human papillomaviruses are associated with many human diseases (Table 7.1) but only types 6, 11, 16, 18, 31, 33 and 35 are regularly associated with cervical neoplasia. HPVs 6, 11, 31 and 35 are associated with condylomas accuminas and the mild forms of CIN, whereas HPVs 16, 18 and 33 are associated with severe CIN and carcinoma of the cervix. The proportion of CIN samples containing HPV is variably reported (Table 7.2) [9, 19, 28–38]. There is also variation between reported studies in the incidence of HPV in squamous cell carcinoma of the cervix (Table 7.3) [9, 19, 20, 30, 32, 33, 35, 39, 40]. The proportion of cervical cancers associated with HPV16 is greater than those associated with HPV18 and differs according to the geographical origin of the tumour. HPV18 appears to be uncommon in cervical tumours from the UK. Not all carcinomas are positive for HPV but it is possible that as more types of HPV are discovered the proportion HPV positivity will increase further. First reports indicated that apparently normal cervical biopsies did not contain HPV16 or 18, but recently DNA–DNA hybridisation studies have shown that 11.5% of normal female cervices were positive for HPV [41]. In these cases the cervices had been defined as normal by cytological, histological and colposcopic methods so it appears that there is a low rate of clinically inapparent infection. Eighteen per cent of women who gave a past history of genital warts

Table 7.1 Human papillomavirus associations with disease

Disease	Associated HPV types
Epidermodysplasia verruciformis	3,5,7,8,10,14,15,17,19,20,21,22,23,24, 25 & 36
Skin cancers arising from epidermo-dysplasia verruciformis	5,8,12,14,19,20,21,22 & 23
Skin papillomas	1,2,3,4,7 & 10
Genital papillomas	6,11 & 16
Bowenoid papillosis	16 & 18
CIN	6,11,16,18,31,33 & 35
Cervical carcinoma	16,18 & 33
Vulvar carcinoma	16,18
Penile carcinoma	16,18
Anal carcinoma	16
Laryngeal papillomas	6,11
Laryngeal carcinoma	16

or had a partner with penile warts but had normal cervices were positive for HPV [42].

Table 7.2 Percentage of CIN samples containing HPV

Reference	Country of origin tissue	Grade of CIN	HPV6	HPV6/11	HPV11	HPV16	HPV18
Durst 1983 [9]	W Germany	I & II III		40 55.6		40.0 44.0	
McCance [28]	UK	I II III (normal)	62.5 60 66 33				
Wagner 1984 [29]	W Germany	I & II III (normal)		18 33 11		33 68 0	
Boshart 1984 [30]	W Germany	All (normal)					0 0
Wickenden 1985 [31]	UK	All	10				
Scholl 1985 [32]	UK	All (normal)				75 0	
McCance 1985 [33]	UK	I II III (normal)	46 20 25 0			55 66 71 18	
Prakash 1985 [19]	Panama	All				66	
Crum 1986 [34]	USA	All		0		83	
Millan 1986 [35]	UK	II/III (normal)			8 0	43 33	18 33
Pater 1986 [36]	Canada	I II III				0 23 50	23 20 26
Jenkins 1986 [37]	UK	I II III				33 33 60	
Campion 1986 [38]	UK	I	46			39	

Table 7.3 Incidence of HPV in squamous cell carcinoma of the cervix (expressed as a percentage)

Reference	Country of origin of tissue	Site of tissue	Cell type	HPV6	HPV11	HPV16	HPV16/18	HPV18	HPVs 6, 8 9, 10 & 11
Durst 1983 [9]	W. Germany	Cervix	Not recorded			61.1			72.2
	Kenya & Brazil	Cervix	Not recorded			34.8			43.5
	W. Germany	Vulva	Not recorded			28.6			42.9
Boshart 1984 [30] No. 5	Africa & Brazil	Cervix	Not recorded					25	
	W. Germany	Cervix	Not recorded					15	
Schneider 1985 [39]	W. Germany	Cervix	Not recorded			50			
Scholl 1985 [32]	U.K.	Cervix	Squamous			45			
			Adeno Ca			0			
			Normal			0			
McCance 1985 [33]	U.K.	Cervix	Squamous	0		92			
			Normal	0		18			
Prakash 1985 [19]	Panama	Cervix	Not recorded			92			
Lancaster 1986	Peru	Cervix	Squamous			61			
Millan 1986 [35]	U.K.	Cervix	Squamous		0	33		0	
			Normal		0	33		33	
McNab 1986 [20]	U.K.	Cervix	Squamous			38		0	
			Adeno Ca			100		6	
		Vulva	Squamous			81		9	

Although this evidence suggests that women with cervical neo-plasia have a significantly higher incidence of HPV infection, epidemiological data are incomplete and a controlled population study, assessing the significance of co-variable risk factors such as sexual behaviour and smoking, is required.

HPV genome organisation

Papillomaviruses are now considered to be a separate family of viruses from the papovavirus group. The virus capsid is approximately 55 nm in diameter and contains circular double-stranded DNA genomes about 8000 bp in length. The DNA is enclosed in an icosahedral capsid containing the virus protein L1 and L2. There are over 50 different types of human papilloma virus now known and all have been de-tected using DNA–DNA hybridisation techniques since HPV cannot be cultured in the laboratory. The different HPV DNA types are iden-tified by their ability to partially cross hybridise at low stringency but individual types are distinguished by having less than 50% cross hybridisation at high stringency [43].

The DNA sequence of HPV1, 6 and 16 have been completely de-termined and HPV18 has been partially sequenced. Because HPVs cannot be propagated in cell culture, much of our knowledge of the virus's molecular biology has come from drawing analogies with bovine papillomaviruses. The organisation of the HPV genome is apparently similar to that of BPV (bovine papillomavirus). The genes can be divided into two groups, early genes encoding for products synthesised before viral DNA replication and late genes encoding for products made after viral DNA synthesis. Presently eight early genes have been identified. The two late genes code for proteins present in the papillomavirus capsid [44] (Fig. 7.1).

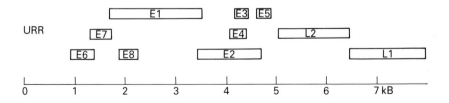

Fig. 7.1   Schematic representation of bovine papillomavirus genome.

Papillomavirus DNA in tumours and tumour cell lines

Papillomaviruses persist and replicate in the cell nucleus. In the pre-invasive cervical and vulvar intraepithelial neoplasias HPV exists separately from cellular DNA, as an episome. There is as yet no indication of the importance of specific sites of integration or association with any particular chromosome [45]. In contrast, in squamous cell carcinomas, originating from several different organs, HPV is integrated into the cellular DNA [46, 47]. Some tumour samples do contain episomal HPV in addition to HPV integrated into the cellular DNA. The importance of this is unclear but could be explained by the observation that tumour samples may contain areas of dysplasia as well as invasive carcinoma so giving rise to the episomal HPV. The integration of HPV into cellular DNA most frequently involves the disruption of the E1–E2 orfs although disruption of L1–L2 has been described. This pattern of disruption of HPV means that only a few early genes are transcribed [45, 47].

Established cell lines have been found to contain HPV (Table 7.4) [4, 48, 49, 50, 51] and are used to study the pattern of integration and gene expression. The most frequent pattern of integrated HPV described so far is a tandem arrangement with HPV DNA separated by a region of cellular DNA. These flanking sequences, which vary according to cell line, are amplified in equivalent proportion to the number of HPV copies per cell. cDNAs show that transcription crosses from the viral DNA into the cellular flanking region. No significant homology of the flanking sequences with known sequences in gene sequence data bases has been demonstrated [52]. In Hela cells one of

Table 7.4 HPV and established cell lines

Cell line	Associated HPV	Copy no. per cell
Hela [48]	18	10–50
SW756 [48]	18	10–50
C 1–4 [48]	18	1
SKG-1 [49]	18	1–2
SKG-11 [49]	18	1–2
CaSki [50]	16	100+
Siha [50]	16	10
SKG-111b [49]	16	1–2
QC-M [51]	16	
QC-U [51]	16	

the integration sites for HPV18 is located upstream from the c-*myc* locus on chromosome 8 [53]. Factors transcribed from integrated HPV sequences might act as a cellular proto-oncogenes to alter the rate of their expression and effect the regulation of cellular growth.

The DNA of HPV present in tumours and cell lines can show considerable re-arrangement (Table 7.5) [47, 54–58]. It is unclear whether this re-arrangement of HPV DNA is important in producing and maintaining the malignant phenotype. It is also not known if the cell lines studied which have been through many hundreds of passages, have suffered alterations to their HPV DNA in culture.

Table 7.5   Some HPV re-arrangements in neoplasia and cell lines

Neoplasia	Size of episomal HPV	Size of integrated HPV	Pattern of re-arrangements
CIN [54]	7.9 kb		None
VIN [55]	16 kb		Dimer of HPV16 with deletion in NCR
Cervical carcinoma [56]		7.9 kb	None
		Sub molar units	Virus/cell junctions
Cervical carcinoma [57]	7.9 kb	7.9 kb	None
Anal carcinoma [47]	7.9 kb	7.9 kb	
	10.7 kb		Duplication of E7, E1 and parts of E6 & E2
Laryngeal carcinoma [48]	7.9 kb	7.9 kb	None
		18 kb	Multiple duplication of E4 and parts of E2, E5, L1 & L2
Cell lines			
Hela [48, 58]			Deleted E2, E4, E5, L1 & L2 region
C44.1 [48, 58]		4.5 kb	
SW756 [48, 58]		7.9 kb	None
CaSki [58]		7.9 kb	None
Siha [58]		5.6 kb	Deleted E2, E4 & E5

Papillomavirus RNA and proteins in tumour cell lines

The E1 protein in Hela cells (HPV18) is 70 kd in size. The role of E1 in BPV is to maintain the episomal state [59]. Sequence homology studies of this protein show similarities to ATPase and nucleotide binding sites, perhaps suggesting an involvement in DNA replication [60].

The part of the genome from 0–800 on the gene map is called the upstream regulatory region (URR). Much of the transcription of mRNA of papillomavirus starts in this region. The product of the E2 orf acts on the URR, stimulating transcription enhancer activity there [61, 62].

The E4 protein is 10 kd in size in CaSki cells and may have a role in virus particle maturation. E6 is of particular interest since it is one of the transforming genes of BPV and thus might be important in a contribution of HPV to tumourgenesis. The E5 orf is present in HPV16 and 18. Both E5 and E6 of BPV1 will transform mouse cells and such transformed cells are tumourgenic in animals [63, 64, 65]. In HPV18 E6 and E7 can transform cells in culture [78]. The E6 protein is 11 kd in size and is translated from a spliced mRNA [66].

In all cell lines the most abundant protein is E7. The E7 protein is cytoplasmic and is approximately 15 kd in HPV16 associated cell lines and 12 kd in HPV18 associated cell lines. In BPV, the E7 protein maintains the replication of the episome at a high copy number [59].

RNA transcription of HPVs has only been studied in tumour cell lines. The genes transcribed in Hela cells (HPV18) are restricted to E6, E6* (a spliced product of E6), E7 and the 5′ end of E1 [52]. CaSki (HPV16) cells transcribe E4, E7, E6 and two spliced versions of E6. Several groups are analysing cDNAs of HPV mRNAs to determine the structures of HPV genes.

Human papillomavirus antibodies

Technical problems have prevented any large scale evaluation of the HPV antibody status of women with cervical neoplasia. As HPV cannot be cultured it is difficult to obtain sufficient quantities of viral antigens to which antibodies can be raised. Owing to the large number of HPV types and the types specific association with disease, the antibody derived may not be sufficiently specific to be of value. Baird has used antibody of broad type specificity against virus particles from BPV2 and found that 60% of women with CIN and 93% with carcinoma of the cervix had detectable antibodies compared with only 15% amongst matched controls [67].

The above problems may soon be circumvented by using modern molecular biology methods. cDNAs corresponding to HPV proteins can be inserted into bacterial or viral expression vectors which will allow the production of large quantities of relevant polypeptides or proteins. These may then be used to raise antibodies that may be more type specific and allow more relevant seroepidemiological studies to be performed. Synthetic peptides may also be useful in providing HPV type specific antibodies since they can be restricted to small antigenic regions which might be type specific.

Papillomaviruses and co-factors in cancer

There is circumstantial evidence that papilloma viruses require co-factors to produce malignant change. Epidermodysplasia verruciformis is a rare skin disease that is frequently associated with HPV infection. Approximately 30% of patients with this disease will develop skin cancers arising from the benign lesion. HPV5 and HPV8 are predominantly associated with this development, but it has also been noted that malignant change only occurs in areas exposed to sunlight so implicating UV irradiation as a co-factor [5,6].

Co-factors are also important in the development of papillomavirus related squamous cell carcinoma of the upper alimentary canal in cattle. Papillomatosis will develop in cattle infected with BPV but malignant transformation to squamous cell carcinoma occurs predominantly in those cattle fed on bracken [68,69]. Bracken contains not only possible chemical carcinogens but also immunosuppressive agents [70,71]. It is, therefore, possible that squamous cell carcinoma in bracken grazing cattle develop as a result of the interaction between BPV and a chemical carcinogen in an immunosuppressed animal. Azothroprine (an immunosuppressive agent), quercetin (a possible chemical carcinogen found in bracken) [72] and BPV4 have been administered singularly or in combination to calves in an experimental attempt to induce squamous cell carcinomas of the upper alimentary tract [73].

There has, as yet, been no direct link between cervical neoplasia and any other co-factor, apart from HPV, but some women with CIN or multifocal intraepithelial neoplasia appear to be immunosuppressed. A reduced level of helper T lymphocytes (T4) and a raised level of suppressor-cytotoxic T lymphocytes (T8) is found systemically in women with multifocal intraepithelial neoplasia [74]. A similar picture is seen in the cervix of women with CIN but their systemic lymphocyte counts (T4/T8) are normal [75]. Many of the constituents of seminal plasma are known to be immunosuppressive but as yet there is little experimental evidence implicating them in cervical neoplasia [76].

CONCLUSIONS

The development of cervical neoplasia is a multistage process. All cervical malignancies pass through some degree of pre-neoplastic change before becoming invasive carcinoma. There is, therefore, a possibility that more than one factor is involved in the malignant transformation of the cervix. Epidemiological evidence shows that the risk of developing cervical cancer is related to sexual behaviour and so a sexually transmissable agent may be involved. Human papillomavirus infections of the genital tract are common and are predominantly caused by HPV6, 11, 16, 18, 31, 33 and 35. In the UK, cervical neoplasia is most frequently associated with HPV16.

Currently, our knowledge of the molecular biology of HPV is limited and many of its properties at present are deduced from comparisons with BPV. Subgenomic fragments of HPV will transform cell lines [49] and these contain the E6 E7 orfs. The E5 and E6 products of BPV will transform cells *in vitro* and cause tumours in nude mice. Despite this ability to transform cells, studies of other diseases linked with papillomavirus infection suggest that alternative factors are required to produce the full malignant phenotype. It is possible that a second factor in cervical neoplasia is the integration of HPV into the cellular genome. The effect of this could be to disrupt the normal control of HPV gene transcription so elevating levels of transforming genes. Alternatively, novel virus-cellular products could be transcribed which act to help produce the malignant phenotype. The integration of HPV would also disrupt cellular genes. If these genes were responsible for cellular growth then disruption or alteration of the product could lead to abnormal cellular growth. At present there is no evidence that HPV is integrated at a specific chromosomal site.

Cigarette smoking increases the chance of developing cervical neoplasia and products of smoking have been detected in the cervix but the mechanism of the interaction between HPV and the products of smoking are poorly understood [77]. Other factors that may be involved include immunosuppression in the woman, either locally or systemically, and interaction between HPV and other viral infections such as HSV2 or CMV.

Human papillomavirus fulfills the general criteria for an oncogenic virus but this does not necessarily prove a causal role in the natural development of a human tumour. Case controlled studies have demonstrated a strong link between HPV and cervical neoplasia. The majority of cervical neoplasias contain HPV DNA whereas approximately 30% of normal cervices are infected with HPV. The true prevalence of HPV infection in the general female population is at present unknown but there is increasing evidence that HPV infection is more common than is apparent in case studies. A high prevalence of HPV infection does not preclude a role for HPV in cervical malignancy but suggests that other events or co-factors are important in cervical neoplasia. This requirement for other events or co-factors pertains to other oncogenic viruses. Infection with hepatitis B virus or Epstein–Barr virus is common in certain parts of the world yet only a few infected people develop the associated malignancy, primary hepatocellular carcinoma with Hepatitis B and Burkitt's lymphoma or undifferentiated nasopharyngeal carcinoma with Epstein–Barr virus. This suggests that infection with an oncogenic virus may be important but other steps are critical for full malignant transformation. It seems likely that infection of the cervix with human papillomavirus, a virus which is known to be sexually transmitted; highly associated with cervical malignancy, and with transforming properties, plays an important role in the aetiology of cervical neoplasia.

REFERENCES

1 Lenoir, G.M. and Bornkamm, G.W. In: Klein, G. (ed.) *Advances in Viral Oncology*. New York: Raven Press 1987, **7**: 173–206.
2 de The, G. Epidemiology of Epstein–Barr virus and associated diseases in man. In: Roizman, B. (ed): *The Herpes Viruses*. New York: Plenum Press, 1982, 25–103.
3 Beasley, R.P., Hwang, L-Y., Lin, C.C. and Chien, C.C. Hepatocellular carcinomas and hepatitis B virus: a prospective study of 22707 men in Taiwan. *Lancet*. 1981, **2**: 1129–1132.
4 Ratner, L., Sarin, P.S., Wong-Staal, F. and Gallo, R.C. Human and primate T-lymphotropic retroviruses (HTLV and PTLV): subtypes, biological activity and role in neoplasia. In: Rigby, P.W.J. and Wilkie, N.M. (eds): *Viruses and Cancer*. Cambridge: Cambridge University Press, 1985, 261–290.
5 Orth, G., Favre, M., Breitburd, F., *et al.* Epidermodysplasia verruciformis: a model for the role of papillomaviruses in human cancer. *Cold Spring Harbor Symp Quant Biol*. 1980, **7**: 259–282.
6 Orth, G. Epidermodysplasia verruciformis: a model for understanding the oncogenicity of human papillomaviruses. In: Evered, D. and Clark, S. (eds)

Papillomaviruses. CIBA Foundation Symposium. Chichester: Wiley, 1986, 157–169.

7 Alexander, E.R. Possible aetiologies of cancer of the cervix other than herpes virus. *Cancer Res.* 1973, **33**: 1485–1496.

8 Schachter, J., Hill, E.C., King, E.B., Heilbronn, D.C., Ray, R.M., Margolis, A.J. and Greenwood, S.A. Chlamydia trachomatis and cervical neoplasia. *JAMA.* 1982, **248**: 2134–2138.

9 Durst, M., Gissmann, L., Ikenberg, H, and zur Hausen, H.A. Papillomavirus DNA from a cervical carcinoma and its prevalence in cancer biopsy samples from different geographic regions. *Proc Natl Acad Sci USA.* 1983, **80**: 3812–3816.

10 Parent-Duchatlet, A.J.B. De la prostitution dans la ville de Paris. *Establissement Encyclographique (Brussels).* 1837, 80–83.

11 Kessler, I.I. Natural history and epidemiology of cervical cancer with special reference to the role of herpes gentialis. In: McBrien, D.C.H. and Slater, T.F. (eds) *Cancer of the Uterine Cervix.* London: Academic Press, 1984, 31–40.

12 Martin, C.E. Martial and coital factors in cervical cancer. *Am J Pub Health.* 1969, **57**: 803–814.

13 Buckley, J.D., Harris, R.W.C., Doll, R., Vessey, M.P. and Williams, P.T. Case control study of the husbands of women with dysplasia or carcinoma of the cervix uteri. *Lancet.* 1981, **2**: 1010–1014.

14 Martinez, I. Relationship of squamous cell carcinoma. *Am J Pub Health.* 1967, **57**: 803–814.

15 Graham, S., Priore, R., Graham, M., Browne, R., Burnett, W. and West, D. Genital cancer in wives of penile cancer patients. *Cancer.* 1979, **44**: 1870–1874.

16 Campion, M.J., Singer, A., Clarkson, P.K. and McCance, D.J. Increased risk of cervical neoplasia in consorts of men with penile condylomata acuminata. *Lancet.* 1985, **1**: 943–946.

17 Aurelian, L., Kessler, I.I., Rosenhein, N.B. and Barbour, G. Viruses and gynecologic cancers: herpes virus protein (ICP-10/AG-4) a cervical tumour antigen that fulfills the criteria for a marker of carcinogenicity. *Cancer.* 1981, **48**: 455–471.

18 Eglin, R.P., Sharp, F., MacLean, A.B., Macnab, J.C.M., Clements, J.B. and Wilkie, N.M. Detection of RNA complementary to herpes simplex virus DNA in human cervical squamous cell neoplasms. *Cancer Res.* 1981, **41**: 3597–3603.

19 Prakash, S.S., Reeves, W.C., Sisson, G.R. *et al.* Herpes simplex virus type 2 and human papillomavirus type 16 in cervicitis, dysplasia and invasive cervical carcinoma. *Int J Cancer.* 1985, **35**: 51–57.

20 Macnab, J.C.M., Walkinshaw, S.A., Cordiner, J.W. and Clements, J.B. Human papillomavirus in clinically and histologically normal tissue of patients with genital cancer. *N Eng J Med.* 1986, **315**: 1052–1058.

21 Galloway, D.A., Copple, C.D. and McDougall, J.K. Analysis of viral DNA sequences in hamster cells transformed by herpes simplex virus type 2. *Proc Natl Acad USA.* 1980, **77**: 880–884.

22 Rawls, E.W., Tompkins, W.A.F., Figuerora, M.E. and Melnick, J.L. Herpesvirus type 2: association with carcinoma of the cervix. *Science.* 1968, **167**: 1255–1256.

23 Rawls, E.W., Clark, A., Smith, K.O., Docherty, J.J., Gilman, S.C., and Graham,

S. Specific antibodies to herpes simplex virus type 2 among women with cervical cancer. In: Essex, M., Todaro, G. and zur Hausen, H. (eds) *Viruses in Naturally Occurring Cancers*. New York: Cold Spring Harbor, 1980, 117–120.

24 Vonka, V., Kanka, J., Hirsch, I. *et al*. Prospective study on the relationship between cervical neoplasia and herpes simplex type-2 virus II. Herpes simplex type-2 antibody presence in sera at enrolment. *Int J Cancer*. 1984, **33**: 61–66.

25 Meisels, A. and Fortin, R. Condylomatous lesions of the cervix and vagina. I Cytological patterns. *Acta Cytol (Baltimore)*. 1976, **20**: 505–509.

26 Purola, E. and Savia, E. Cytology of gynecologic condyloma acuminata. *Acta Cytol (Baltimore)*. 1977, **21**: 26–31.

27 Ferenczy, A., Braun, L. and Shah, K.V. Human papillomavirus (HPV) in condylomatous lesions of cervix: a comparative ultrastructure and immunohistochemical study. *Am J Surg Pathol*. 1981, **5**: 661–670.

28 McCance, D.J., Walker, P.G., Dyson, J.L., Coleman, D.V. and Singer, A. Presence of human papillomavirus DNA sequences in cervical intraepithelial neoplasia. *Br Med J*. 1983, **287**: 784–788.

29 Wagner, D., Ikenberg, H., Boehm, N. and Gissmann, L. Identification of human papilomavirus in cervical swabs by deoxyribonucleic acid *in situ* hybridisation. *Obstet Gynecol*. 1984, **64**: 767–772.

30 Boshart, M., Gissmann, L., Ikenberg, H., Kleinheinz, A., Scheurlen, W. and zur Hausen, H. A new type of papillomavirus DNA, its presence in genital cancer biopsies and in cell lines derived from cervical cancer. *EMBO J*. 1984, **3**: 1151–1157.

31 Wickenden, C., Steele, A., Malcolm, A.D.B. and Coleman, D.V. Screening for wart virus infection in normal and abnormal cervices by DNA hybridisation of cervical scrapes. *Lancet*. 1985, **1**: 65–67.

32 Scholl, S.M., Kingsley Pillers, E.M., Robinson, R.E. and Farrell, P.J. Prevalence of human papillomavirus type 16 DNA in cervical carcinoma samples in East Anglia. *Int J Cancer*. 1985, **35**: 215–218.

33 McCance, D.J., Clarkson, P.K., Dyson, J.L., Walker, P.G. and Singer A. Human papillomavirus types 6 and 16 in multifocal intraepithelial neoplasias of the female lower genital tract. *Br J Obstet Gynaecol*. 1985(b), **92**: 1093–1100.

34 Crum, C.P., Nagai, N., Levine, R.U. and Silverstein, S. *In situ* hybridisation analysis of HPV16 DNA sequences in early cervical neoplasia. *Am J Pathol*. 1986, **123**: 174–182.

35 Millan, D.W.M., Davies, J.A., Torbet, T.E. and Campo, M.S. DNA sequences of human papillomavirus types 11, 16 and 18 in lesions of the uterine cervix in the west of Scotland. *Br Med J*. 1986, **293**: 93–96.

36 Pater, M.M., Dunne, J., Hogan, G., Ghatage, P. and Pater, A. Human papillomavirus types 16 and 18 sequences in early cervical neoplasia. *Virology*. 1986, **155**: 13–18.

37 Jenkins, D., Tay, S.K., McCance, D.J., Campion, M.J., Clarkson, P.K. and Singer, A. Histological and immunocytochemical study of cervical intraepithelial neoplasia (CIN) with associated HPV6 and HPV16 infections. *J Clin Pathol*. 1986, **39**: 1177–1180.

38 Campion, M.J., McCance, D.J., Cuzick, J. and Singer A. Progressive potential of mild cervical atypia: prospective cytological, colposcopic, and virological study. *Lancet*. 1986, **2**: 237–240.

39 Schneider, A., Karus, H., Schuhmann, R. and Gissmann, L. Papillomavirus infection of the lower genital tract: detection of viral DNA in gynecological swabs. *Int J Cancer*. 1985, **35**: 443–448.

40 Lancaster, W.D., Castellano, C., Santos, C., Delgrado, G., Kurman, R.K. and Jenson, A.B. Human papillomavirus deoxyribonucleic acid in cervical carcinoma from primary and metastatic sites. *Am J Obstet Gynaecol*. 1986, **154**: 115–119.

41 Troon, P.G., Arrand, J.R., Wilson, L.P. and Sharp, D.S. Human papillomavirus infection of the uterine cervix of women without cytological signs of neoplasia. *Br Med J*. 1986, **293**: 1261–1264.

42 McCance, D.J., Campion, M.J., Clarkson, P.K., Jenkins, D. and Singer, A. Prevalence of human papillomavirus type 16 DNA sequences in cervical intraepithelial neoplasia and invasive carcinoma of the cervix. *Br J Obstet Gynaecol*. 1985(a). **92**: 1101–1105.

43 Pfister, H., Krubke, J., Dietrich, W., Iftner, T. and Fuche, P.G. Classification of the papillomaviruses—mapping the genome. In: Evered, D. and Clark, S. (eds) *Papillomaviruses*. CIBA Foundation Symposium, Chichester: Wiley, 1986, 3–14.

44 Pilacinski, W.P., Glassman, D.L., Krzyzek, R.A., Sadowski, P.L. and Robbins, A.K. Cloning and expression in *Escherichia coli* of the bovine papillomavirus L1 and L2 open reading frames. *Biotechnology*. 1984, **1**: 356–360.

45 Gissman, L., and Schwarz, E. Persistence and expression of human papillomavirus DNA in genital cancer. In: Evered, D. and Clark, S. (eds) *Papillomaviruses*. Ciba Foundation Symposium. Chichester: Wiley, 1986, 190–197.

46 Durst, M.M., Kleinheinz, A., Hotz, M. and Gissmann, L. The physical state of human papillomavirus type 16 DNA in benign and malignant tumours. *J Gen Virol*. 1985, **66**: 1515–1522.

47 Scheurlen, W., Stremlau, A., Gissman, L., Hohn, D., Zenner, H-P. and zur Hausen, H. Rearranged HPV16 molecules in anal and in a laryngeal carcinoma. *Int J Cancer*. 1986, **38**: 671–676.

48 Schwarz, E., Freese, U.K., Gissmann, L., Mayer, W., Roggenbuck, B., Stremlau, A. and zur Hausen, H. Structure and transcription of human papillomavirus sequences in cervical carcinoma cells. *Nature*. 1985, **314**: 111–114.

49 Tsunokawa, Y., Takebe, N., Kasamatsu, T., Terada, M. and Suimura, T. Transforming activity of human papillomavirus type 16 DNA sequences in a cervical cancer. *Proc Natl Acad Sci USA*. 1986(a), **83**: 2200–2203.

50 Yee, C., Krishnan-Hewlett, I., Baker, C.C., Schlegel, R. and Howley, P.M. Presence and expression of human papillomavirus sequences in human cervical carcinoma cell lines. *Am J Pathol*. 1985, **119**: 361–366.

51 Shirasawa, H., Tomita, Y., Sekiya, S., Takamizawa, H. and Simizu, B. Integration and transcription of human papillomavirus type 16 and 18 sequences in cell lines derived from cervical carcinomas. *J Gen Virol*. 1987, **68**: 583–591.

52 Schneider-Gadicke, A. and Schwarz, E. Different human cervical carcinoma cell lines show similar transcription patterns of human papillomavirus type 18 early genes. *EMBO J*. 1986, **5**: 2285–2292.

53 Durst, M., Croce, C.R., Gissmann, L., Schwarz, E. and Huebner, K. Papillomavirus sequences integrate near cellular oncogenes in some cervical carcinomas. *Proc Natl Acad Sci USA*. 1987, **84**: 1070–1074.

54 Durst, M., Schwarz, E. and Gissmann, L. Integration and persistence of human papillomavirus DNA in genital tumours. In: Peto, R. and zur Hausen, H. (eds) *Viral Etiology of Cervical Cancer* (Banbury Report). New York: Cold Spring Harbor, 1986, **2**: 1430–1431.

55 Kennedy, I.M., Simpson, S., MacNab, J.C.M. and Clements, J.B. Human papillomavirus type 16 DNA from a vulvar carcinoma *in situ* is present as head-to-tail dimeric episomes with a deletion in the non-coding region. *J Gen Virol.* 1987, **68**: 451–462.

56 Durst, M., Kleinheinz, A., Hotz, and Gissmann, L. The physical state of human papillomavirus type 16 DNA in benign and malignant tumours. *J Gen Virol.* 1985, **66**: 1515–1522.

57 Smotkin, D. and Wettstein, F.O. Transcription of human papillomavirus type 16 early genes in a cervical cancer and a cancer-derived cell line and identification of the E7 protein. *Proc Natl Acad Sci USA.* 1986, **83**: 4680–4684.

58 Pater, M.M. and Pater, A. Human papillomavirus types 16 and 18 sequences in carcinoma cell lines of the cervix. *Virology.* 1985, **145**: 313–318.

59 Lusky, M. and Botchan, M.R. Genetic analysis of the bovine papillomavirus type 1 trans-acting replication factors. *J Virology.* 1985, **53**: 955–965.

60 Clertant, P. and Seif, I. A common function for polyoma virus large T and papillomavirus E1 protein. *Nature.* 1984, **311**: 276–279.

61 Androphy, E.J., Lowy, D.R. and Schiller, J.T. Bovine papillomavirus E2 trans-activating gene product binds to specific sites in papillomavirus DNA. *Nature.* 1987, **325**: 70–73.

62 Haugen, T.H., Cripe, T.P., Ginder, D.G., Karin, M. and Turek, L.P. Trans-activation of an upstream early gene promoter of bovine papillomavirus-1 by a product of the viral E2 gene. *EMBO J.* 1987, **6**: 145–152.

63 Schiller, J.T., Vass, W.C. and Lowy, D.R. Identification of a second transforming region in bovine papillomavirus DNAP. *Proc Natl Acad Sci USA.* 1984, **81**: 7880–7884.

64 Yang, Y-C., Okayama, H. and Howley, P. Bovine papillomavirus contains multiple transforming genes. *Proc Natl Acad Sci USA.* 1985, **82**: 1030–1034.

65 Schiller, J.T., Vass, W.C., Vousden, K.H. and Lowry, D.R. E5 open reading frame of bovine papillomavirus type 1 encodes a transforming gene. *J Virol,* 1986, **57**: 1–6.

66 Seedorf, K., Oltersdorf, T., Drammer, G, and Rowekamp, W.Identification of the early proteins of human papillomavirus type 16 (HPV 16) and type 18 (HPV 18) in cervical carcinoma cells. *EMBO J.* 1987, **6**: 139–144.

67 Baird, P.J. Serological evidence for the association of papillomavirus and cervical neoplasia. *Lancet.* 1983, **2**: 17–18.

68 Jarrett, W.F.H., McNeil, P.E. Grimshaw, W.T.R., Selman, I.E. and McIntyre, W.I.M. High incidence of cattle cancer with a possible interaction between an environmental carcinogen and a papillomavirus. *Nature.* 1978(a). **274**: 215–217.

69 Jarrett, W.F.H., Murphy, J., O'Neill, P.E. and Laird, H.M. Virus-induced papillomas of the alimentary tract of cattle. *Int J Cancer.* 1978(b), **22**: 323–328.

70 Evans, A., Prorok, J.H., Cole, R.C., *et al.* The carcinogenic, mutagenic and teratogenic toxicity of bracken. *Proc R Soc Edinb B (Biol Sci).* 1982, **81**: 65–67.

71 Evans, W.C., Patel, M.C. and Koohy, Y. Acute bracken poisoning in homogastric and ruminant animals. *Proc R Soc Edinb B (Biol Sci)*. 1982, **81**: 29–64.

72 Pamucku, A.M., Yalchiner, S., Matcher, J.F, and Bryant, G.T. Quercetin, a rat intestinal and bladder carcinogen present in bracken fern (*Pteridium Aquilinum*). *Cancer Res*. 1980, **20**: 3468–3472.

73 Campo, M.S. and Jarrett, W.F.H. Papillomavirus infection in cattle: viral and chemical cofactors in naturally occurring and experimentally induced tumours. In: Evered, D. and Clark, S. (eds) *Papillomaviruses*. CIBA Foundation Symposium. Chichester: Wiley, 1986, 117–131.

74 Carson, L.F., Twiggs, L.B., Fukushima, M., Ostrow, M.S., Faras, A.J. and Okagaki, T. Human genital papilloma infections: an evaluation of immunological competence in the genital papilloma syndrome. *Am J Obstet Gynaecol*. 1986, **155**: 784–789.

75 Tay, S.K., Jenkins, D., Maddox, P. and Singer, A. Lymphocyte phenotypes in cervical neoplasia and human papillomavirus infection. *Br J Obstet Gynecol*. 1987, **94**: 16–21.

76 James, K. and Hargreave, T.B. Immunosuppression by seminal plasma and its possible clinical significance. *Immunol Today*. 1984, **5**: 357–363.

77 Sasson, I.M., Haley, N.J., Hoffmann, D., Wynder, E.L., Hellberg, D. and Nilsson, S. Cigarette smoking and neoplasia of the uterine cervix: smoke constituents in cervical mucus. *New Engl J Med*. 1985, **312**: 315–316.

78 Bedell, M.A. Jones, K.M. and Laimins L.A. The E6-E7 region of human papillomavirus type 18 is sufficient for transformation of NIM 3T3 and Rat-1 cells. *J Virol*. 1987, **61**: 3635–3640.

8 STEROID HORMONE RECEPTOR STRUCTURE AND FUNCTION

J.O. WHITE

THE CELLULAR response to steroid hormones is mediated, at least in part, by specific intracellular receptor proteins. Following ligand binding, these receptors become activated to forms with increased affinity for nuclear structures and this results in the modulation of expression of target genes.

The precise mechanism that allows the steroid receptor to interact with its target genes is the subject of active research employing the modern techniques of cellular and molecular biology. Recently, as a result of the application of these modern techniques several aspects of the structure and function of steroid receptor complexes have been re-investigated or explored for the first time. These include the subcellular localisation of receptor, the subunit composition of receptor, the domain structure of hormone receptors and the nature of the steroid hormone responsive DNA elements. Each of these has a bearing on the understanding of the mechanisms of hormone action and potential implications for the control of hormone dependent cancer. In this chapter, these recent advances will be discussed.

THE SUBCELLULAR LOCALISATION OF THE STEROID RECEPTOR

It is used to be thought that steroid receptors were cytoplasmic, translocating to nucleus after steroid hormone binding. In subcellular preparations from tissues exposed *in vivo* to relatively low concentrations of hormone it was found that steroid receptors behaved as soluble cytosolic proteins. Following steroid stimulation the majority of the steroid receptors are recovered in the nuclear fraction. The translocation hypothesis of steroid receptor transfer to the nucleus following hormonal stimulation was developed to accomodate these observations [1]. Recently, using immunohistochemical or cell enucleation techniques which lead to minimal disruption of normal cellular architecture, it has been demonstrated that the receptors for oestradiol, progesterone and glucocorticoids are nuclear associated proteins [2,3,4,5]. Two forms of receptor with differing affinities for nuclear structures have been proposed. The unliganded receptor with lower affinity for nuclear structures is thought to become soluble during tissue disruption while the higher affinity forms, induced by ligand binding, remain associated with the nucleus [6]. Exposure to steroid *in vivo* may change the relative proportion of these two forms of receptor resulting in differential partitioning during subcellular fractionation and hence an apparent decrease in receptor in the cytosolic fraction following hormone stimulation. Autoradiographic studies of the subcellular distribution of labelled steroid combined with immunohistochemistry now provides compelling evidence that steroid hormone receptors are nuclear associated proteins [2]. However, the cellular mechanisms that determine the nucleocytoplasmic segregation of proteins remain to be established [7].

Steroid hormone receptor status assessment in tumours arising in steroid responsive tissues has previously relied on determinations made on cytosolic preparations [8]. If cytosolic receptor is a preparation artefact then it is more relevant to assess nuclear receptor status. Evidence in support of the clinical value of nuclear receptor determination in cancers already exists [9], where disease free interval and response to hormonal therapy is significantly improved in patients whose tumours contain 'functional' receptor, i.e. receptor distributed in the soluble and nuclear fractions.

The coexistence of the progresterone receptor, an oestrogen regulated protein, with the oestradiol receptor indicates an increased likelihood of hormone responsiveness [10]. It is suggested that the presence of the progesterone receptor reflects tissue responding to oestradiol and assumes receptor regulation is similar in cancer cells to normal tissues. There are several reports that support this assumption [11,12,13,14]. Although the redistribution of receptors during homogenisation may lead to localisation artefact, their presence in the cytosolic fraction remains of potential clinical benefit. Qualitative differences in cytosol receptors, based on binding to artificial nuclear matrices which may reflect aspects of nuclear and biological function *in vivo*, provide further prognostic and therapeutic information [15].

RECEPTOR SUBUNIT COMPOSITION

Cytosolic steroid hormone receptors prepared from tissues and cells not previously exposed to steroid stimulation exist as oligomeric structures of molecular weight 250 000–300 000 [16]. Exposure to steroid activates receptor, a process which confers increased affinity for nuclei and DNA, and which is accompanied by a decrease in molecular size and net charge [17,18,19,20].

In many studies, the possibility of non-specific protein association resulting from the receptor becoming soluble during tissue preparation cannot be ruled out. This has led to doubts regarding the relevance to the *in vivo* situation of the observation of aggregated forms of receptor and of the subunit dissociation that accompanies steroid induced activation *in vitro* [21]. However, evidence in support of receptor activation being a physiologically relevant event involving subunit dissociation *in vivo* has been presented [22,23]. Hence, investigation of the subunit composition of steroid hormone receptor complexes *in vitro* may provide information pertinent to the molecular mechanisms involved in receptor activation to forms with increased nuclear affinity.

Oliogmeric non-activated forms of the receptors for progesterone, oestrogen, androgen and glucocorticoids contain a non-hormone binding 90 000 molecular weight phosphoprotein [24]. This antigen is not associated with the steroid binding unit of the progesterone and glucocorticoid receptor following activation [22, 25]. The 90 000 molecular weight non-hormone binding unit associated with non-activated receptors represents as much as 1% of total cellular protein and has been demonstrated to be indistinguishable from a major heat-shock stress protein (HSP) [26]. The presence of the HSP in the oligomeric form of the progesterone receptor has been demonstrated both in purified preparations and in the absence of agents used to stabilise cytosol complexes [27], evidence which is presented in favour of a non-artefactual association. The presence of this protein in nuclei has led to the suggestion of its involvement in regulating the conversion of the low affinity receptor to one with a higher affinity for DNA [27]. Studies of the cellular response to hormonal stimulation at physiological and non-physiological temperatures [28] may contribute to an understanding of the role of HSP in receptor function.

Stress proteins are also found in non-stressed cells and may be involved in the cellular response to external stimuli. The synthesis of HSP is sensitive to glucocorticoids [29] and is regulated during cellular differentiation [30]. Recent evidence indicates that the non-hormone binding 90 000 molecular weight protein that forms complexes with steroid binding proteins is indistinguishable from a 90 000 molecular weight protein that forms complexes with the Rous sarcoma virus transforming protein pp60 v-*src* [31], and other tyrosine kinase oncogene products [32]. When complexed with this protein the tyrosine kinase activity of pp60 v-*src* is repressed [33]. A possible role, therefore, of HSP is in the modulation of protein kinase activity and the state of phosphorylation of steroid receptors. The oestradiol receptor contains phosphotyrosine residues [34] and the progesterone receptor is an excellent substrate for the tyrosine kinase activity associated with growth factor receptors [35]. Kinase activity has been demonstrated to co-purify with the progesterone receptor [36] and a role for receptor phosphorylation/dephosphorylation in regulating steroid binding and receptor activation has been discussed [37,38,39,20]. Given the role of phosphorylation as a major cellular regulatory mechanism [40], it is a reasonable proposal that steroid effector proteins should be modulated in such a manner. It may be excessive, based on available evidence, to speculate that the role of a cellular homologue of an oncogene product is to modify the biological function of steroid receptors and that a heat-shock protein is involved in modulating this process. However in the context of searching for the role of proto-oncogenes and how their functions may differ from the oncogenic product, it is an attractive working hypothesis, especially as oncogene products are already implicated as modifiers of normal cellular signal transduction.

An alternative explanation of the regulation of the oligomeric form of the oestrogen receptor is provided by the observation that the partially purified protein contains an intrinsic serine protease activity that is responsible for mediating the ligand-induced increase in receptor affinity for isolated nuclei [41]. It is suggested that specific peptide cleavage, either of the steroid-binding unit itself or of a non-steroid-binding protein subunit may facilitate dissociation of the oligomeric structure. Limited proteolysis of the steroid receptor, by endogenous or exogenous enzyme, leading to the the generation of functional forms capable of binding to nuclei or DNA has previously been reported [16,42,43].

If indeed aggregated receptor represents the non-activated species and disaggregated receptor represents a species at some point in the pathway leading to the biologically functional state, one might expect to observe a functional correlate of this. In human breast cancer, therefore, the molecular forms of the oestrogen receptor were deter-

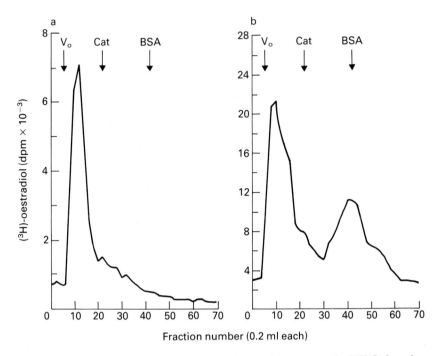

Fig. 8.1   Resolution of oestrogen receptor in human breast cancer by HPLC. Samples were resolved using a spherogel-TSK G 3000 SW column at a flow rate of 0.6 ml/min in 10 mM phosphate, 1 mM DTT, 20% (v/v) glycerol pH 7.4. Vo = void volume. Cat = catalase, BSA = bovine serum albumin.

mined and compared with the concentration of the progesterone receptor which is an oestrogen sensitive gene product. The oestradiol receptor, measured by high performance size exclusion liquid chromatography, was found to be a high molecular weight (300 000) protein sometimes found in association with a 60 000 molecular weight protein (Fig. 8.1). Examination of the concentration of the progesterone receptor according to the resolvable forms of the oestrogen receptor revealed a significantly higher concentration in tumours containing the lower molecular weight species (Fig. 8.2). Tumours containing the lower molecular weight species also contained receptors with a greater capacity to bind to olio(dT)-cellulose which is a measure of receptor activation [44]. The nature of the proteins [45,46,47,48] and other macromolecules [49,50] that are associated with steroid

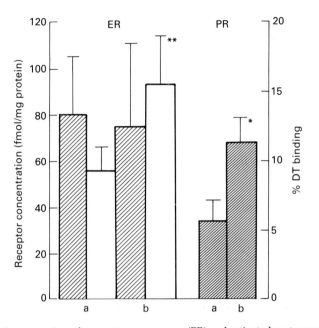

Fig. 8.2   Concentration of progesterone receptor (PR) and activated oestrogen receptor (ER). PR in ER positive samples that were resolved as (a) 300K or (b) 300K+60K. ER concentration (hatched) and percentage binding to oligo(dT)-cellulose (open bars). Significantly different from (a), *$P < 0.001$, **$P < 0.025$ (t test).

receptors and their role, if any, in the cellular response to hormonal stimulation, remains under investigation.

THE MOLECULAR BIOLOGY OF STEROID RECEPTORS

Steroid receptors represent a minor proportion of total cellular proteins in hormone responsive cells and the messenger RNAs encoding these receptors are a relatively minor abundance class. However, by applying the techniques of molecular biology the cDNAs for the glucocorticoid [51,52], oestradiol [53,54,55,56,57] and progesterone [58,59,60] receptors have now been cloned. This has represented a major advance in our understanding of the structure and function of steroid hormone receptors, as analysis of the nucleotide sequence of the cloned cDNA has allowed the amino acid sequence of these receptors to be deduced. This new information has already allowed description of certain functional characteristics common to these effector proteins and it has been elegantly shown that expression of transfected receptor genes is sufficient to confer hormone sensitivity on previously unresponsive cells [61,62,63].

The DNA-binding domain

Sequence comparisons between the glucocorticoid, oestradiol and progesterone receptors [64] have defined two conserved regions that have functionally important domains. The DNA-binding domain is a highly conserved 66 amino acid sequence rich in cysteine residues spanning amino acids 185–251 of the human oestrogen receptor, 581–647 of the chicken progesterone receptor and 421–487 of the human glucocorticoid receptor. This cysteine, arginine and lysine rich domain is potentially capable of forming 'finger regions', stabilised by co-ordinate binding of a zinc molecule to cysteine residues, which could interact with the major groove of the DNA [65,59,55,66]. There is also good biochemical evidence to suggest that the basic amino acids arginine and lysine are functional residues in the interaction of steroid receptors with polyanionic artificial nuclear matrices [67]. Repeated units containing Cys-Arg-Lys rich sequences were first observed in the structure of the Xenopus transcription factor TF III A [68] and have been since found in a number of other nucleic acid-binding proteins [69].

Deletion of amino acids 132–198 or 199–264 of the oestrogen receptor almost completely abolishes its nuclear association [70]. Conversely, expression of amino acids 407–566 in a mutant glucocorticoid receptor is sufficient to retain its ability to interact with specific glucocorticoid response elements [71]. Point and insertional mutations affecting the putative DNA-binding finger of the oestrogen and glucocorticoid receptors [51,65,72] prevent their activation of marker genes. Such mutations do not affect the steroid binding capacity of the respective receptors. Thus, the integrity of the cysteine, arginine and lysine rich region of the oestradiol and glucocorticoid receptor seems to be essential for their recognition of, and interaction with, specific DNA sequences in the genes under their control.

The homology between the putative DNA-binding region of the oestradiol receptor and that of the glucocorticoid and progesterone receptor is of the order of 50–60%. The glucocorticoid and progesterone receptors are approximately 90% homologous in this region [64, 56]. It has been proposed that the conserved amino acids in this region of steroid receptors are responsible for the core structure, including the DNA-binding fingers. The variable amino acids in this domain may confer the specificity of receptor interaction with regulatory elements of the target gene.

Comparative hydropathicity studies, which indicate the hydrophobic and hydrophilic regions within a given amino acid sequence of the putative DNA-binding domain of the oestradiol, progesterone and glucocorticoid receptors, reveal identical profiles [56]. This suggests even greater conservation of secondary or tertiary structure in this region of the receptors.

Thus, there are amino acid motifs which are conserved in proteins capable of interacting with nucleic acids. What, therefore, are the unique features of the steroid receptors that determine the specificity of gene regulation? Experiments using a chimaeric receptor generated by replacing the 66 amino acid DNA-binding region of the oestrogen receptor with that of the human glucocorticoid receptor provide some insights into this question [72]. This chimaeric receptor, when transiently expressed in HeLa cells is capable of binding oestradiol but cannot activate an oestradiol-responsive gene that is sensitive to activation by the wild type oestrogen receptor. However, the chimaeric receptor, containing the glucocorticoid receptor DNA-binding domain, activates a glucocorticoid reponsive gene and requires the presence of oestradiol to do so. The wild type oestrogen receptor does not stimulate expression of the glucocorticoid responsive gene. The conclusion from these experiments is that the specificity of receptor-gene interaction is determined by the DNA-binding domain of the receptor. The conserved amino acids in the DNA-binding domain of all steroid receptors are thought to provide a broad structural framework within which the variable amino acids dictate specificity.

That a chimaeric receptor is capable of activating a glucocorticoid responsive gene in the presence of oestradiol suggest that those structural features essential for communication between the steroid and DNA-binding domains are retained. A sequence of amino acids whose predicted secondary structure would confer a flexibility in receptor structure that might accomodate contact between two functional domains in the oestradiol receptor has been described [55]. Similarly, a putative hinge region linking the DNA- and steroid-binding domains of the glucocorticoid receptor has been demonstrated to be necessary for transcriptional activation [65]. Insertional mutations in this region generate a receptor with dexamethasone binding similar to the wild type receptor but with diminished capacity for transcriptional activation of a glucocorticoid sensitive gene. These mutations are thought to inhibit the allosteric transformation necessary for ligand induction of activation of the DNA-binding domain. It is generally assumed that the hormone-binding domain interacts with the DNA-binding domain during ligand-induced receptor activation [18,73]. The hinge region of the oestradiol and glucocorticoid receptor may provide such flexibility but the nature of the interaction between the two domains remains to be established. Given the homology between the DNA-binding domains of the oestradiol and glucocorticoid receptors it has been suggested that conserved regions of the ligand-binding domain are involved in this site–site interaction [51]. Comparison of the carboxy-terminal region of the oestradiol and glucocorticoid receptors reveals a sequence of 29 amino acids, 18 of which are identical [51]. A model has, therefore, been proposed in which a loop formed by these conserved amino acids would mask the DNA-binding domain. Steroid binding would alter the conformation of this loop and hence unmask the DNA-binding domain. The intervening region between the DNA-binding and steroid-binding domains of the oestradiol and glucocorticoid receptors show little homology. The secondary structure of this region and the conformation it may impose could provide a further determinant of specificity in receptor structures and the nature of their interaction with chromatin.

The hormone-binding domain

The hormone-binding domain of the oestradiol, glucocorticoid and progesterone receptors have been mapped to the carboxy-terminal. Hydroplotting suggests a hydrophobic region which may form a binding-pocket for steroid. The requirement of these regions in the glucocorticoid and oestradiol receptor for ligand binding has been established in mutation experiments that parallel those which established the function of the DNA-binding domain. The homology between the steroid-binding domains of the steroid receptors is numerically less striking than the corresponding homology between the DNA-binding domains [64]. Interestingly, however, there is a high conservation of amino acid residues (52%) in the ligand-binding region of the progesterone and glucocorticoid receptors, two receptors with similar although not identical steroid specificity.

Recent reports describing *in vitro* interaction of the glucocorticoid and progesterone receptors with their specific DNA-binding sites in the absence of cognate steroid, raised the possibility of receptors having constitutive activity [74]. Contrary reports of the requirement of dexamethasone for transcriptional activity *in vivo* point to the potential relaxation of constraints on receptor function following *in vitro* isolation [75]. However, the ability of glucocorticoid receptor mutants to be transcriptionally active in the absence of dexamethasone *in vivo* indicates the potential for the constitutive activity of truncated receptor species [71]. This, of course, has significant implications for hormone dependent cancer as the apparent absence of detectable receptors on the basis of lack of hormone binding may conceal the presence of a mutated receptor that is biologically active in the absence of its cognate ligand. A precedent for truncated receptors lacking their hormone-binding domain is provided by the description of homology of the v-*erb*B oncogene product with the intracellular domain of the epidermal growth factor receptor but lacking the extracellular ligand binding site.

Homology of receptors with oncogene products

Sequence comparisons between the oestrogen, glucocorticoid and progesterone receptors and that of the product of the v-*erb*A gene of the avian erythroblastosis virus reveal significant homologies [58,53,55,60,56]. The similarities are most striking in the DNA-binding region and to a lesser extent in the steroid-binding domain. These homologies between hormone receptors and v-*erb*A suggested that v-*erb*A, and possibly its cellular homologue c-*erb*A, may be hormone-binding proteins capable of regulating specific gene expression.

Cloning of c-*erb*A and characterisation of its protein product as the thyroid hormone receptor has recently been reported [76,77]. Interestingly, the v-*erb*A gene product does not bind thyroid hormone and it is likely that the viral product has lost its hormone-binding capacity as a result of mutation [76]. Whether gene regulation by v-*erb*A and c-*erb*A is similar remains unclear. However, as discussed above, there are now several precedents for gene regulation by receptors defective in their ligand-binding domains. Thyroid hormone induces a variety of metabolic effects and is involved in tissue specific differentiation. The identification of a cellular homologue of a viral oncogene product as the receptor for such a regulatory hormone may suggest that the oncogenic potential of v-*erb*A is related to its inappropriate constitutive regulation/deregulation of cellular differentiation genes. V-*erb*A is not itself oncogenic but potentiates the transformation of cells transfected with v-*erb*B, v-*src*, v-*fps* or v-*sea*, allowing erythroblasts to grow in an independent fashion [78].

An interesting feature of the similarity of hormone receptor proteins with the v-*erb*A oncogene product is the possibility that they have evolved from a common primordial gene and represent a family of regulatory proteins that influence gene transcription [64]. The divergence in their structure may have arisen to accommodate the more complex biology of eukaryotic systems. A family of *erb*A proto-oncogenes has been described and their genes located to chromosomes 3 and 17 [76]. This raises the intriguing possibility that distinct forms of receptors may exist in normal cells which display qualitatively different responses to hormonal stimulation.

Other functional domains of steroid receptor

In addition to the DNA- and steroid-binding domains of steroid receptors, two other regions have been described that are necessary for receptor mediated transcription of glucocorticoid responsive genes. Mutations in the amino terminal region of the glucocorticoid receptors at positions 120, 204 and 214 result in receptors with steroid-binding affinity similar to the wild type but diminished transcriptional activity. This domain of the glucocorticoid receptor, termed tau-1, coincides with the major immunogenic domain [65] and may be the fragment which is missing in 'increased nuclear transfer' nt^i variants of the glucocorticoid receptor. The nt^i receptor binds to specific DNA sequences with decreased affinity but to non-specific DNA with a higher affinity [79]. Comparison of the N-terminal region of steroid receptors reveals very low homology which may indicate that the information for receptor-specific regulation of transcription resides within this region. Deletion of the first 106 amino acids of the N-terminal domain of the mouse glucocorticoid receptor resulted in a functional receptor confirming that the N-terminal transcription regulatory functions are closer to the DNA-binding domain [51]. The second functional domain of the glucocorticoid receptor, described as tau-2 [65], corresponds to the hinge region between the DNA and steroid-binding domains discussed above. Interestingly, a single amino acid change in the corresponding region of the v-*erb*A transforming protein completely abolishes its biological activity [78].

ACTIVATED OESTROGEN RECEPTORS AND IMPLICATIONS FOR BREAST CANCER

The binding of oestradiol to its receptor leads to receptor activation increasing its affinity for nuclei, DNA and artificial nuclear matrices [80,17,44]. The *in vitro* assays of receptor activation employing polyanionic matrices, including DNA and oligo(dT)-cellulose provide an indication of the alteration in surface charge that may accompany steroid-induced conformational changes during activation [81]. However, these *in vitro* assays distinguish only the capacity of the receptor to bind to DNA and do not provide information concerning specificity. Results from model systems indicate that glucocorticoid and oestradiol receptors which are deficient in their ability to interact with DNA are a phenotype of cells resistant to hormonal control [79]. In the case of the glucocorticoid receptor the genetic background to the receptor mutant with reduced DNA-binding ability has been attributed to a single amino acid substitution, arginine 484 to histidine in the DNA-binding domain [51].

It is possible, therefore, that receptors with apparently normal steroid binding capacity could be heterogenous with respect to other functional domains and hence be deficient in biological activity. In order to investigate this possibility in human breast cancer, oestrogen receptor steroid binding capacity and ability to bind to oligo(dT)-cellulose, which has similar properties to DNA cellulose [82], has been examined [15,83,84]. In oestrogen receptor positive tumours obtained from premenopausal women, oligo(dT)-binding was observed in 44 out of 83 specimens. In postmenopausal subjects the corresponding figure was 133 out of 190 (p < 0.005) [15]. This in itself is an interesting observation given the poorer prognosis of premenopausal breast cancer patients.

One hundred and forty seven patients with stage I-III disease, in whom the only postoperative treatment was radiotherapy for nodal involvement, were evaluated for disease recurrence and then categorised according to receptor status. Segregation of patients according to positivity of the oestrogen receptor revealed no significant effect on the proportion remaining free of disease (Fig. 8.3). However, on subdivision of oestrogen receptor positive patients into activated (oligo(dT)-cellulose binding) and non-activated (failed to bind to oligo(dT)-cellulose) groups, a highly significant difference became apparent (Fig. 8.3, Table 8.1). Thus the prognosis for patients whose

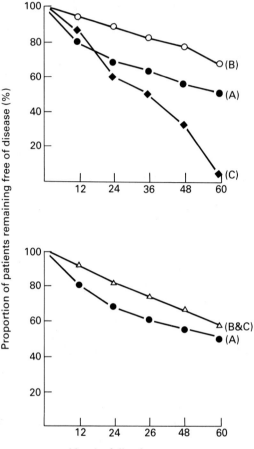

Fig. 8.3 Disease recurrence and receptor status. Proportion of patients remaining disease free according to oestrogen receptor (ER) status. A = negative; B = activated ER; C = non-activated ER.

tumours contained activated oestrogen receptor is better than for patients whose tumours contained non-activated receptor or were receptor negative. Further support for the biological significance of the distinction between activated and non-activated receptor is provided by the difference in creatine kinase activity and progesterone receptor incidence, between each oestrogen-sensitive protein [10,85] (Table 8.2).

The preceeding description of the functional domains of steroid hormone receptors and their possible association with non-receptor

Table 8.1   Disease recurrence and activated oestrogen receptor (ER)

Months after surgery	ER activated		ER non-activated		ER neg	
	N	R	N	R	N	R
0–12	63	3	21	3	63	12
13–24	60	4	17	5	49	7
25–36	46	3	12	2	36	3
37–48	33	2	6	2	23	2
49–60	16	2	1	1	12	1

At the indicated intervals following surgery the number of patients at risk (N) and the number of recurrences (R) were noted. The differences between each phenotype were analysed by the log rank test:
ER activated significantly different from ER non-activated chi square $= 5.05, P < 0.025$.
ER activated significantly different from ER negative chi square $= 13.76, P < 0.0005$.

subunits, provide intriguing explanations of the possible reasons for lack of oestrogen receptor binding to oligo(dT)-cellulose in certain breast tumours. The following suggestions may obviously have parallels in other steroid receptors and the tumours in which they occur. Firstly, mutation within the DNA-binding domain itself or between this domain and the steroid binding domain may alter the conformational change required for interaction with DNA. It would be interesting, therefore, to compare the relative capacity and affinity of steroid hormone receptors derived from normal and tumour tissues to bind to the specific responsive elements of target genes. Secondly, the subunit composition of the steroid receptors may be altered such that the non-steroid-binding units persisitently mask the DNA-binding

Table 8.2   Comparison of creatine kinase (CK) and progesterone receptor (PR) incidence according to the presence or absence of activated oestrogen receptor (ER). Significantly different from non-activated ER. * $= P < 0.02$ Mann Whitney 'U' test, and † $= P < 0.05$ chi square

ER	CK (mU/mg protein)	PR (incidence)
Activated	61.0* (12–488) $n = 40$	103/133†
Non-activated	38.9 (10.5–433) $n = 29$	37/57

domain of the steroid receptor. This could reflect changes in stoichiometry of the subunit components or modification of these proteins that may alter their functional interaction.

Evidence obtained from the rat uterus indicates that oestrogen receptor activation is preferentially stimulated by GTP [44]. Nucleotide analogues which do not act as phosphate donors were also capable of activating the oestrogen receptor, thus suggesting that nucleotide-binding rather than phosphate donation may be important. A nucleotide-binding site distinct from the DNA-binding site has recently been demonstrated for the oestrogen receptor [86]. Modulation of the activity of nucleotide-binding proteins as a result of ADP-ribosylation, catalysed by the transferase activity of microbial enzymes is well documented [87]. Cholera toxin catalyses the transfer of ADP-ribose, using NAD as co-factor, to the guanidinium group of arginine. This covalent substitution modifies the biological activity of the retinal rod protein transducin and of the adenyl cyclase complex [88]. In rat uterine cytosol preparations cholera toxin inhibits oestrogen receptor activation, is dependent on the presence of NAD and has no significant effect on ligand binding (Table 8.3). These data obviously do not demonstrate a direct effect on oestrogen receptor, however, the importance of arginine residues in the DNA-binding domain [51] and the selective effect of cholera toxin (Table 8.3) suggest the possibility of

Table 8.3 Cholera toxin inhibition of receptor activation

	REC (cpm/0.2 ml cytosol)	REC bound to dT	% REC bound to dT
4°C 1h	27159±4553 (7)	6295±1905** (7)	23.05±5.52 (7)
30°C 1h	24393±5834 (12)	13128±3452 (12)	54.18±7.84 (12)
30°C 1h + CT + NAD	24932±6541 (11)	7711±3501* (11)	30.77±10.37 (11)
30°C 1h + CT − NAD	24214±3942 (3)	11360±1500 (3)	47.37±6.09 (3)

Receptor determination and activation was as described in reference number 44. CT = cholera toxin; NAD = nicotinamide adenine dinucleotide. Significantly different from 30°C 1h. * = $P < 0.005$, ** = $P < 0.001$ (t test).

receptor ADP-ribosylation being another level of control of steroid-receptor function.

HORMONE RESPONSE ELEMENTS

Steroid receptors act as transcriptional regulators by interacting in a selective manner with DNA hormone response elements (HRE). These elements act in concert with transcription initiation elements responsible for the binding of RNA polymerase II and the initiation of RNA synthesis. Insertion of these elements can confer hormonal sensitivity upon an otherwise insensitive gene [79].

A common eight nucleotide sequence in the progesterone receptor-binding site of the uteroglobin gene resembles the sequence of DNA sites that interact with the glucocorticoid receptor [88]. The ability of the HRE of the mouse mammary tumour virus (MMTV) to mediate glucocorticod, progestin and androgen induction of gene transcription [89] suggests that the HRE contains binding sites for all three hormone receptors. The homologies in the DNA-binding domains of steroid receptors may explain their ability to recognise common DNA sequences in HRE [90].

The chicken lysozyme gene can be induced by glucocorticoids, progestins and other classes of steroid hormones [91]. Two receptor-binding sites with reciprocal affinities for the glucocorticoid and progesterone receptor have been found adjacent to the promoter sequence [92]. In the hormone regulatory element which has a higher affinity for the progesterone receptor, distinct contact sites for this hormone receptor and the glucocorticoid receptor have been described [91]. This suggests subtle differences in the recognition mechanisms for these two receptors and these are postulated to explain the differential regulation of one gene by different hormones.

Oestradiol does not induce gene transcription in constructs regulated by MMTV DNA [89]. Furthermore, in experiments designed to demonstrate binding of the oestrogen receptor to HRE in the 5' region flanking the vitellogenin A_2 gene [93] it was reported that MMTV DNA does not have specific binding sites for the oestrogen receptor [94]. Differences in the DNA-binding domains of the steroid receptors may conveniently explain the differences between oestradiol on the one hand and progesterone and glucocorticoid on the other with respect to their interaction with MMTV. However, both oestradiol and progesterone are known to induce ovalbumin gene transcription

[95] requiring defined DNA elements upstream of the transcription initiation site [96]. Thus, the conformation adopted by steroid receptors and specifically required for the activation of selected target genes may reflect the properties of only a relatively small number of amino acids.

CONCLUSIONS

Recently, it has been demonstrated that interaction of transcription factors with the inducible promoter of MMTV is stimulated by glucocorticoids [97] possibly as a result of the modification of the binding site for these factors. It is conceivable, therefore, that different steroid receptors induce conformational changes that dramatically alter the accessibility of other protein-binding regulatory sites in nuclear chromatin, as a result of small differences in the manner in which they interact with HRE. The determination of the molecular mechanism of this process, which may include site specific DNA methylation [98] and alteration of nucleoprotein interactions [99,100,101,102] remains to be elucidated. The pertubations of these interactions in cells where there is aberrant expression of cellular proto-oncogenes [103] may represent an initial step leading to profound effects on normal cellular function.

REFERENCES

1 Jensen, E.V. and De Sombre, E.R. Estrogen–receptor interaction. *Science*. 1973, **181**: 126–134.

2 Ennis, B.W., Stumpf, W.E., Gasc, J.M. and Baulieu, E.E. Nuclear localization of progesterone receptor before and after exposure to progestin at low and high temperatures: autoradiographic and immunohistochemical studies of chick oviduct. *Endocrinology*. 1986, **119**: 2066–2075.

3 Fuxe, K., Wikstrom, A.C., Okret, S. *et al*. Mapping of glucocorticoid receptor immunoreactive neurons in the rat tele- and diencephalon using a monoclonal antibody against rat liver glucocorticoid receptor. *Endocrinology*. 1985, **117**: 1803–1812.

4 King, W.J. and Greene, G.L. Monoclonal antibodies localise oestrogen receptor in the nuclei of target cells. *Nature*. 1984, **307**: 745–747.

5 Welshons, W.V., Lieberman, M.E. and Groski, J. Nuclear localisation of unoccupied oestrogen receptor. *Nature*. 1984, **307**: 747–749.

6 Gorski, J., Welshons, W.V., Sakai, D. *et al*. Evolution of a model of estrogen action. *Recent Prog Horm Res*. 1986, **42**: 297–330.

7 De Robertis, E.M. Nucleocytoplasmic segregation of proteins and RNAs. *Cell*. 1983, **32**: 1021–1025.

8 Williams, M.R., Todd, J.M., Ellis, I.O. *et al.* Oestrogen receptors in primary and advanced breast cancer: an eight year review of 704 cases. *Br J Cancer.* 1987, **55**: 67–73.

9 Soutter, W.P. and Leake, R.E. Steroid hormone receptors in gynaecological cancers. In: Bonar, J. (ed) *Recent Advances in Obstetrics and Gynaecology.* 1986, **15**: 175–194.

10 Horwitz, K.B. and McGuire, W.L. Estrogen control of progesterone receptor in human breast cancer. *J Biol Chem.* 1978, **253**: 2223–2228.

11 Eckert, R.L. and Katzenellenbogen, B.S. Physical properties of estrogen receptor complexes in MCF-7 human breast cancer cells. Differences with anti-estrogen and estrogen. *J Biol Chem.* 1982, **257**: 8840–8846.

12 Mullick, A. and Katzenellenbogen, B.S. Progesterone receptor synthesis and degradation in MCF-7 human breast cancer cells as studied by dense amino acid incorporation. Evidence for non-hormone binding receptor precursor. *J Biol Chem.* 1986, **261**: 13235–13243.

13 Philipson, K.A., Elder, M.G. and White, J.O. The effects of medroxyprogesterone acetate on enzyme activities in human endometrial carcinoma. *J Steroid Biochem.* 1985, **23**: 1059–1064.

14 Scholl, S. and Lippman, M.E. The oestrogen receptor in MCF-7 cells: evidence from dense amino acid labelling for rapid turnover and a dimeric model of activated nuclear receptor. *Endocrinology.* 1984, **115**: 1295–1301.

15 White, J.O., Herschman, M.J., Parmar, G., Philipson, K.A., Elder, M.G., Habib, N.A. and Wood, C.B. Activated oestrogen receptor in human breast cancer: clinical and biochemical correlates. *Brit J Surg.* 1987, **74**: 588–590.

16 Sherman, M.R. and Stevens, J. Structure of mammalian steroid receptors: evolving concepts and methodological developments. *Ann Rev Physiol.* 1984, **46**: 83–105.

17 Grody, W.W., Schrader, W.T. and O'Malley, B.W. Activation, transformation and subunit structure of steroid hormone receptors. *Endocr Rev.* 1982, **3**: 141–163.

18 Muller, R.E., Traish, A.M., Hirota, T., Bercel, E. and Wotiz, H.H. Conversion of estrogen receptor from a state with low affinity for estradiol into a state of higher affinity does not require 4S to 5S dimerization. *Endocrinology.* 1985, **116**: 337–345.

19 Sakai, D. and Gorski, J. Estrogen receptor transformation to a high-affinity state without subunit–subunit interactions. *Biochemistry.* 1984, **23**: 3541–3547.

20 Smith, A.C., Elsasser, M.S. and Harmon, J.M. Analysis of glucocorticoid receptor activation by high resolution two-dimensional electrophoresis of affinity-labelled receptor. *J Biol Chem.* 1986, **261**: 13285–13292.

21 King, R.J.B. Receptor structure: a personal assessment of the current status. *J Steroid Biochem.* 1986, **25**: 451–454.

22 Mendel, D.B., Bodwell, J.E., Gametchu, B., Harrison, R.W. and Munck. A. Molybdate-stabilized nonactivated glucocorticoid-receptor complexes contain a 90-kDa non-steroid-binding phosphoprotein that is lost on activation. *J Biol Chem.* 1986, **261**: 3758–3763.

23 Raaka, B.M., Finnerty, M., Sun, E. and Samuels, H.H. Effects of molybdate on steroid receptors in intact GH_1 cells. Evidence for dissociation of an intracel-

lular 10S receptor oligomer prior to nuclear accumulation. *J Biol Chem.* 1985, **260**: 14009–14015.

24 Joab, I., Radanyi, C., Renoir, M. *et al.* Common non-hormone binding component in non-transformed chick oviduct receptors of four steroid hormones. *Nature.* 1984, **308**: 850–853.

25 Sanchez, E.R., Tuft, D.O., Schlesinger, M.J. and Pratt, W.B. Evidence that the 90-kDa phosphoprotein associated with the untransformed L-cell glucocorticoid receptor is a murine heat shock protein. *J Biol Chem.* 1985, **260**: 12398–12401.

26 Catelli, M.G., Binart, N., Jung-Testas, I., Renoir, J.M., Baulieu, E.E., Feramisco, J.R. and Welch, W.J. The common 90-kd protein component of non-transformed '8S' steroid receptors is a heat-shock protein. *EMBO J.* 1985, **4**: 3131–3135.

27 Renoir, J.M., Buchou, T. and Baulieu, E.E. Involvement of a non-hormone-binding 90 kilodalton protein in the non-transformed 8S form of the rabbit uterus progesterone receptor. *Biochemistry.* 1986, **25**: 6405–6413.

28 Wolffe, A.P., Perlman, A.J. and Tata, J.R. Transient paralysis by heat shock of hormonal regulation and gene expression. *EMBO J.* 1984, **3**: 2763–2770.

29 Kassambalides, E.J. and Lanks, K.W. Dexamethasone can modulate glucose-regulated heat shock protein synthesis. *J Cell Physiol.* 1983, **114**: 93–98.

30 Morange, M., Div, A., Bensaude, O. and Babinet, C. Altered expression of heat shock proteins in embryolonal carcinoma and mouse early embryonic cells. *Mol Cell Biol.* 1984, **4**: 730–735.

31 Schuh, S., Yonemoto, W., Brugge, J., Bauer, V.J., Riehl, R.M., Sullivan, W.P. and Toft, D.O. A 90 000 dalton binding protein common to both steroid receptors and the Rous sarcoma virus transforming protein pp60^{v-src}. *J Biol Chem.* 1985, **260**: 14292–14296.

32 Ziemiecki, A., Catelli, M.G., Joab, I. and Moncharmont, B. Association of the heat shock protein HSP90 with steroid hormone receptors and tyrosine kinase oncogene products. *Biochem Biophys Res Commun.* 1986, **138**: 1298–1307.

33 Courtneidge, S.A. and Bishop, J.M. Transit of pp60^{v-src} to the plasma membrane. *Proc Natl Acad Sci USA.* 1982, **79**: 7117–7121.

34 Migliaccio, A., Rotondi, A. and Auricchio, F. Estradiol receptors: phosphorylation on tyrosine in uterus and interaction with anti-phosphotyrosine antibody. *EMBO J.* 1986, **5**: 2867–2872.

35 Woo, D.D.L., Fay, S.P., Griest, R., Coty, W., Goldfine, I.and Fox, C.F. Differential phosphorylation of the progesterone receptor by insulin, epidermal growth factor and platelet-derived growth factor receptor tyrosine protein kinases. *J Biol Chem.* 1986, **261**: 460–467.

36 Garcia, T. Buchou, T., Renoir, J.M., Mester, J. and Baulieu, E.E. A protein kinase copurified with chick oviduct progesterone receptor. *Biochemistry.* 1986, **25**: 7937–7942.

37 Dahmer, M.K., Nousley, P.R. and Pratt, W.B. Effects of molybdate and endogenous inhibitors on steroid receptor inactivation, transformation and translocation. *Ann Rev Physiol.* 1984, **46**: 67–81.

38 Logeat, F., Le Cunff, M., Pamphile, R. and Milgrom, E. The nuclear bound form of the progesterone receptor is generated through a hormone-dependent phosphorylation. *Biochem Biophys Res Commun.* 1985, **131**: 421–427.

39 Migglaccio, A., Rotondi, A. and Auricchio, F. Calmodulin-stimulated phosphorylation of 17B-oestradiol receptor on tyrosine. *Proc Natl Acad Sci USA.* 1984, **81**: 5921–5925.

40 Cohen, P. The role of protein phosphorylation in neural and hormonal control of cellular activity. *Nature.* 1982, **296**: 613–620.

41 Puca, G.A., Abbondanza, C., Nigro, V., Armetta, I., Medici, N. and Molinari, A.M. Estradiol receptor has proteolytic activity that is responsible for its own transformation. *Proc Natl Acad Sci USA.* 1986, **83**: 5367–5371.

42 Sala-Trepat, J.M. and Vallet-Strouve, C. Binding of the oestradiol receptor from calf uterus to chromatin. *Biochem Biophys Acta.* 1974, **371**: 186–202.

43 Wrange, O. and Gustaffson, J.A. Separation of the hormone and DNA-binding sites of the hepatic glucocorticoid receptor by means of proteolysis. *J Biol Chem.* 1978, **253**: 856–865.

44 Myatt, L., Cukier, D., Elder, M.G. and White, J.O. Activation of oestrogen receptor complexes: evidence for the distinct regulation of ligand and oligonucleotide binding sites. *Biochem Biophys Acta.* 1985, **845**: 304–310.

45 Coffer, A.I., Lewis, K.M., Brockas, A.J. and King, R.J.B. Monoclonal antibodies against a component related to soluble oestrogen receptor. *Cancer Res.* 1985, **45**: 3686–3693.

46 Peleg, S., Schrader, W.T., Edwards, D.P., McGuire, W.L. and O'Malley, B.W. Immunological detection of a protein homologous to chicken progesterone receptor B subunit. *J Biol Chem.* 1985, **260**: 8492–8501.

47 Tai, P.K.K., Maeda, Y., Nakao, K.N.G., Duhring, J.L. and Faber, L.E. A 50-kilodalton protein associated with progestin, estrogen, androgen and glucocorticoid receptors. *Biochemistry.* 1986, **25**: 5269–5275.

48 Wrange, O., Carlstedt-Duke, J. and Gustafsson, J.A. Stoichiometric analysis of the specific interaction of the glucocorticoid receptor with DNA. *J Biol Chem.* 1986, **261**: 1177–1178.

49 Kovacic-Milivojevic, B. and Vedeckis, W.V. Absence of detectable ribonucleic acid in the purified, untransformed mouse glucocorticoid receptor. *Biochemistry.* 1986, **25**: 8266–8273.

50 Webb, M.L., Schmidt, T.J., Robertson, N.M. and Litwack, G. Evidence for an association of a ribonucleic acid with the purified unactivated glucocorticoid receptor. *Biochem Biophys Res Commun.* 1986, **140**: 204–211.

51 Danielsen, M., Northrop, P. and Ringold, G.M. The mouse glucocorticoid receptor: mapping of functional domains by cloning, sequencing and expression of wild-type and mutant receptor proteins. *EMBO J.* 1986, **5**: 2513–2522.

52 Hollenberg, S.M., Weinberger, C., Ong, E.S. *et al.* Primary structure and expression of a functional human glucocorticoid receptor cDNA. *Nature.* 1985, **318**: 635–670.

53 Green, S., Walter, P., Kumar, V., Kurst, A., Bornert, J.M., Argos, P. and Chambon, P. Human oestrogen receptor cDNA: sequence, expression and homology to v-erb-A. *Nature.* 1986, **320**: 134–139.

54 Greene, G.L., Gilna, P., Waterfield, M., Baker, A., Hort, Y., Shine, J. Sequence and expression of human estrogen receptor cDNA. *Science.* 1986, **231**: 1150–1154.

55 Krust, A., Green, S., Argos, P., Kumar, V., Walter, P., Bornert, J.M. and

Chambon, P. The chicken oestrogen receptor sequence: homology with v-erb-A and the human oestrogen and glucocorticoid receptors. *EMBO J.* 1985, **5**: 891–897.

56 Maxwell, B.L., McDonnell, D.P., Conneely, O.M., Schulz, T.Z., Greene, G.L. and O'Malley, B.W. Structural organization and regulation of the chicken estrogen receptor. *Mol Endocr.* 1987, **1**: 25–35.

57 Walter, P., Green, S., Greene, G. *et al.* Cloning of the human estrogen receptor cDNA. *Proc Natl Acad Sci USA.* 1985, **82**: 7889–7893.

58 Conneely, O.M., Sullivan, W.P., Toft, D.O. *et al.* Molecular cloning of the chicken progesterone receptor. *Science.* 1986, **233**: 767–770.

59 Jeltsch, J.M., Krozowski, Z., Quirn-Stricker, C. *et al.* Cloning of the chicken progesterone receptor. *Proc Natl Acad Sci USA.* 1986, **83**: 5424–5428.

60 Loosefelt, H., Atger, M., Misrahi, M. *et al.* Cloning and sequence analysis of rabbit progesterone receptor complementary DNAP. *Proc Natl Acad Sci USA.* 1986, **83**: 9045–9049.

61 Druege, P.M., Klein-Hitpas, L., Green, S., Stack, G., Chambon, P. and Ryffel, G.U. Introduction of oestrogen-responsiveness into mammalian cell lines. *Nucleic Acids Res.* 1986, **14**: 9239–9337.

62 Miesfeld, R., Rusooni, S., Godowski, P.J. *et al.* Genetic complementation of a glucocorticoid receptor deficiency by expression of cloned receptor cDNA. *Cell.* 1986, **46**: 389–393.

63 Vanderbilt, J.N., Miesfeld, R., Maler, B.A. and Yamamoto, K.R. Intracellular receptor concentration limits glucocorticoid-dependent enhancer activity. *Mol Endocr.* 1987, **1**: 68–74.

64 Green, S. and Chambon, P. A superfamily of potentially oncogenic hormone receptors. *Nature.* 1986, **324**: 615–617.

65 Giguere, V., Hollenberg, S.M., Rosenfeld, M.G. and Evans, R.M. Functional domains of the human glucocorticoid receptor. *Cell.* 1986, **46**: 645–652.

66 Weinberger, C., Hollenberg, S.M., Rosenfeld, M.G. and Evans, R.M. Domain structure of human glucocorticoid receptor and its relationship to the v-erb-A oncogene product. *Nature.* 1985, **318**: 670–672.

67 Schmidt, T.S. and Litwack, G. Activation of the glucocorticoid-receptor complex. *Physiol Rev.* 1982, **62**: 1131–1192.

68. Miller, J., McLachlan, A.D. and Klug, A. Repetitive zinc-binding domains in the protein transcription factor III A of Zenopus oocytes. *EMBO J.* 1985, **4**: 1609–1614.

69 Berg, J. Potential metal-binding domains in nucleic acid-binding proteins. *Science.* 1986, **232**: 485–487.

70 Kumar, V., Green, S., Staub, A. and Chambon, P. Localisation of the oestradiol-binding and putative DNA-binding domains of the human oestrogen receptor. *EMBO J.* 1986, **5**: 2231–2236.

71 Godowski, P.J., Rusconi, S., Misefeld, R. and Yamamoto, K.R. Glucocorticoid receptor mutants that are constitutive activators of transcriptional enhancement. *Nature.* 1987, **325**: 365–368.

72 Green, S. and Chambon, P. Oestradiol induction of a glucocorticoid-responsive gene by a chimaeric receptor. *Nature.* 1987, **325**: 75–78.

73 Sakai, D. and Gorski, J. Estrogen receptor transformation to a high-affinity state without subunit-subunit interactions. *Biochemistry.* 1984, **23**: 3541–3547.

74 Willmann, T. and Beato, M. Steroid-free glucocorticoid receptor binds specifically to mouse mammary tumour virus DNA. *Nature.* 1986, **324**: 688–691.

75 Becker, P.B., Gloss, B., Schmid, W., Strahle, U. and Schutz, G. *In vivo* protein-DNA interactions in a glucocorticoid response element require the presence of the hormone. *Nature.* 1986, **324**: 686–688.

76 Sap, J., Munoz, A., Damm, K. *et al.* The c-erb-A protein is a high-affinity receptor for thyroid hormone. *Nature.* 1986, **324**: 635–640.

77 Weinberger, C., Thompson, C.C., Ong, E.S., Lebo, R., Gruol, D.J. and Evans, R.M. The c-erb-A gene encodes a thyroid hormone receptor. *Nature.* 1986, **324**: 641–646.

78 Damm, K., Beug, H., Graf, T. and Vennstrom, B. A single point mutation in erb-A restores the ethyroid transforming potential of a mutant avian erythroblastosis virus (AEV) defective in both erb-A and erb-B oncogenes. *EMBO J.* 1987, **6**: 375–382.

79 Yamamoto, K.R. Steroid Receptor Regulated transcription of specific genes and gene networks. *Ann Rev Genet.* 1985, **19**: 209–252.

80 Chong, M.T. and Lippman, M.E. Effects of temperature, nucleotides and sodium molybdate on activation and DNA binding of estrogen, glucocorticoid, progesterone and androgen receptors in MCF-7 human cancer cell lines. *J Recept Res.* 1982, **2**: 575–600.

81 Myatt, L. and Wittliff, J. Characterisation of non-activated and activated estrogen and anti-estrogen complexes by high performance ion exchange chromatography. *J Steroid Biochem.* 1986, **24**: 1041–1048.

82 Thrower, S., Hall, C., Lim, L. and Davison, A.N. The selective isolation of the uterine oestradiol-receptor complex. *Biochem J.* 1976, **160**: 271–280.

83 Fernandez, M.D., Burn, J.I., Sauven, P.D., Parmar, G., White, J.O. and Myatt, L. Activated oestrogen receptors in breast cancer and response to endocrine therapy. *Eur J Cancer Clin Oncol.* 1984, **20**: 41–46.

84 Myatt, L., White, J.O., Fernandez, M.D. and Burn, J.J.I. Human breast tumour cytosol oestrogen receptor binding to oligo(9dT)-cellulose. *Br J Cancer.* 1982, **45**: 964–967.

85 Kaye, A.M., Hallowes, R., Cox, S. and Sluyser, M. Hormone responsive creatinine kinase in normal and neoplastic mammary glands. *Ann NY Acad Sci.* 1986, **464**: 218–230.

86 Hutchens, T.W., Li, C.H. and Bersch, P.K. Urea-induced transformation of native oestrogen receptor and evidence for separate DNA- and ATP-binding sites. *Biochem Biophys Res Commun.* 1986, **139**: 1250–1255.

87 Ueda, K. and Hayaishi, O. ADP-ribosylation. *Annu Rev Biochem.* 1985, **54**: 73–100.

88 Bailly, A., Le Page, C., Rauch, M. and Milgrom, E. Sequence specific DNA binding of the progesterone receptor to the uteroglobin gene: effects of hormone, antihormone and receptor phophorylation. *EMBO J.* 1986, **5**: 3235–3241.

89 Cato, A.C.B., Henderson, D. and Ponta, H. The hormone response element of the mouse mammary tumour virus DNA mediates the progestin and androgen induction of transcription in the proviral long terminal repeat region. *EMBO J.* 1987, **6**: 363–368.

90 Cato, A.C.B., Miksicek, R., Schutz, G., Arnemann, J. and Beato, M. The

hormone regulatory element of a mouse mammary tumour virus mediates progesterone induction. *EMBO J.* 1986, **5**: 2237–2240.

91 Ahe, Von der, D., Renoir, J.M., Buchou, T., Baulieu, E.E. and Beato, M. Receptors for glucocorticosteroid and progesterone recognize distinct features of a DNA regulatory element. *Proc Natl Acad Sci USA.* 1986, **83**: 2817–2821.

92 Ahe, Von der, D., Janich, S., Scheidereit, C., Renkawitz, R., Schutz, G. and Beato, M. Glucocorticoid and progesterone receptors bind to the same sites in two hormonally regulated promotors. *Nature.* 1985, **313**: 706–709.

93 Klein-Hitpass, L., Schorpp, M., Wagner, U. and Ryffel, G.U. An oestrogen-responsive element derived from the 5′ flanking region of the Xenopus vitellogenin A2 gene functions in transfected human cells. *Cell.* 1986, **46**: 1053–1061.

94 Weisz, A., Coppola, L. and Bresciani, F. Specific binding of estrogen receptor to sites upstream and within the transcribed region of the chicken ovalbumin gene. *Biochem Res Commun.* 1986, **139**: 396–402.

95 O'Malley, B.W., Schwartz, R.J. and Schrader, W.T. A review of regulation of gene expression by steroid hormone receptors. *J Steroid Biochem.* 1976, **7**: 1151–1159.

96 Dean, D.C., Cope, R., Knoll, B.J., Riser, M.E. and O'Malley, B.W.O. A similar 5′-flanking region is required for estrogen and progesterone induction of ovalbumin gene expression. *Nature.* 1984, **305**: 551–554.

97 Cordingley, M.G., Riegel, A.T. and Hager, G.L. Steroid-dependent interaction of transcription factors with the inducible promotor of mouse mammary tumour virus *in vivo*. *Cell.* 1987, **48**: 261–270.

98 Saluz, H.P., Jiricny, J. and Jost, J.P. Genomic sequencing reveals a positive correlation between the kinetics of strand-specific DNA demethylation of the overlapping estradiol/glucocorticoid-receptor binding sites and the rate of avian vitellogenin mRNA synthesis. *Proc Natl Acad Sci USA.* 1986, **83**: 7167–7171.

99 Hora, J., Horton, M.J., Toft, D.O. and Spelsberg, T.C. Nuclease resistance and the enrichment of native nuclear acceptor sites for the avian oviduct progesterone receptor. *Proc Natl Acad Sci USA.* 1986, **83**: 8839–8843.

100 Kaufmann, S.H., Okret, S., Wilkstrom, A.C., Gustafsson, J.A. amd Shaper, J.H. Binding of the glucocorticoid receptor to the rat liver nuclear matrix. The role of disulfide bond formation. *J Biol Chem.* 1986, **261**: 1162–1167.

101 Kirsch, T.M., Miller-Diener, A. and Litwack, G. The nuclear matrix is the site of glucocorticoid receptor complex action in the nucleus. *Biochem Biophys Res Commun.* 1986, **137**: 640–648.

102 Singh, R.K., Ruh, M.F., Butler, W.B. and Ruh, T.S. Acceptor sites on chromatin for receptor bound by estrogen versus anti-estrogen in anti-estrogen-sensitive and resistant MCF-7 cells. *Endocrinology.* 1986, **118**: 1087–1095.

103 Jaggi, R., Salmons, B., Muellener, D. and Groner, B. The v-mos and H-ras oncogene expression represses glucocorticoid hormone-dependent transcription from the mouse mammary tumour virus LTR. *EMBO J.* 1986, **5**: 2609–2616.

9 BIOLOGICAL APPROACHES TO CANCER THERAPY

K. SIKORA

R EMARKABLE advances in molecular biology over the last two decades have resulted in a considerable increase in our understanding of malignant transformation in experimental systems and insights into the mechanisms of the growth disorder that result in human cancer. The interaction of tumour with host is complex. Over the last 100 years evidence has been obtained for an immune response as well as a range of other responses which may control tumour growth under certain circumstances. The very growth of a tumour, however, indicates that restraining mechanisms have failed in a patient with cancer.

The new technology of molecular biology has given rise to a revolution in pharmacology. Our ability to isolate, clone and express specific genes using recombinant DNA technology has resulted in the production of pharmaceutical quantities of highly purified molecules. Complex mixtures of proteins can be dissected into their constituent components and used for carefully controlled clinical trials. It may be possible by the judicious use of a purified biological agent to correct the abnormality that led to cancer and indeed reverse it. Biological agents may therefore have profound significance in both the prevention and treatment of cancer.

Gene cloning became a reality in the late 1970s. Clinical trials with genetically engineered proteins are still in their infancy. The pace of acquisition of new products is staggering and is driven by the highly competitive commercial environment of biotechnology. In this chapter, I will consider the interferons as a model system in which the greatest experience of biological agents has been gained and then review some other, and perhaps more promising biological approaches to the treatment of cancer. The potential of monoclonal antibodies as diagnostic and therapeutic agents has already been considered in Chapter 6.

THE INTERFERONS

Interferon (IFN) was discovered in 1957 by Isaacs and Lindeman following the observation that cells infected with virus were protected from simultaneous infection with a second virus [1]. Initially, IFN was believed to be a single molecule. IFN consists of a whole family of molecules with similar biological properties. Many of the actions of IFN are species specific. When examined more closely the IFN system can be shown to have diverse effects, not only on the intracellular metabolism of target cells but also on the immune system. Given the ever increasing complexity of this system it is hardly surprising that 20 years of laboratory work were required before serious clinical trials could begin.

Structure

The complete purification and understanding of the structure of the IFN gene family has only recently been achieved, although some details still remain to be resolved. Standard chemical techniques have allowed the separation of the major related groups. The nomenclature is extremely confusing and continues to undergo changes as more information is gleaned [2]. There are three major families of human interferon produced by leucocytes, fibroblasts and lymphocytes (Table 9.1). IFN was firstly purified by thiocyanate precipitation and gel exclusion chromatography from these three sources and used as an antigen to immunise animals. The antibodies so produced were found

Table 9.1   The interferons—nomenclature

Family	Species	Comment
Hu IFNα	Hu IFNα (PIF)	α Partially purified leucocyte
	Hu IFNα Leu	α Leucocyte
	Hu IFNα Lym	α Lymphoblastoid
	Hu IFNα N	α Namalwa cell lymphoblastoid
	Hu IFNα 2A	α Clone A recombinant
	Hu IFNα 2B	α Clone B recombinant
	Hu IFNα A/D	α Clone A/D recombinant
Hu IFNβ	Hu IFN β1	β clone recombinant
Hu IFNγ	Hu IFN γ1	γ clone recombinant

to distinguish the different types of IFN. A major problem is that the different sources of IFN do not necessarily produce IFN of one type.

Stimulated leucocytes produce both alpha and gamma IFN. Type 1 and type 2 IFN (Table 9.2) can be distinguished by antibodies raised against preparations that are thought to be pure. Stability at low pH is a characteristic of leucocyte and fibroblast IFN but not that produced by mitogen or antigen stimulated lymphocytes.

Table 9.2 The interferons—properties

Leucocyte lymphoblastoid	Fibroblast	Immune
Viral induced	Viral induced	Antigen induced Mitogen induced
Type 1	Type 1	Type 2
pH2 stable	pH2 stable	pH2 unstable
Not glycosylated	Glycosylated	Glycosylated
At least 17 genes	At least 2 genes	Single gene
No introns	Introns (except β)	Introns
On chromosome 9	Dispersed on chromosomes 2,5,9.	On chromosome 12

There was considerable confusion for some years as to whether different interferon types would glycosylate or not. It is now clear that alpha interferon is not glycosylated. Despite increases in the sophistication of biochemical techniques such as electrophoresis and chromatography it took the advent of gene cloning to allow the complete structural relationships of the IFNs to be understood. It is also clear that there are more related molecules yet to be isolated. Their structure will no doubt be determined over the next few years.

It is the ability to isolate specific pieces of human DNA and to expand them into limitless quantities in bacteria that has enabled the rapid and detailed analysis of the structure of IFN. To clone for IFN genes, leucocytes were triggered into a high production rate by a combination of viral infection and superinduction by metabolic inhibitors. RNA was extracted from these cells. It was known that the RNA coding for interferon sedimented as 12S on ultracentrifugation. Using this technique, it was possible to achieve partial purification and enrichment of IFN mRNA. These mRNAs were used as templates for the production of cDNA by the enzyme reverse transcriptase. The cDNA copies were inserted into plasma vectors which were in turn replicated in bacteria. Many genes were thus incorporated into the bacteria but few coded for IFN. The resulting cDNA library can be amplified and maintained indefinitely. By a process of screening and elimination IFN clones were isolated. Once one sequence was found which coded for IFN; hybridisation techniques were used to identify other cDNA clones in the library which contained homologous sequences.

DNA known to code for IFN can be labelled to high specific activity with p32 nucleotides. This labelled probe was used to identify clones in the library that hybridised to it. These clones were isolated and expanded and their relationship to the probe DNA ascertained. The technique has been made much simpler with the discovery of rapid DNA sequencing techniques which enable large fragments of DNA to be sequenced precisely [3].

The first cloning of IFN cDNA was reported in 1980. Two DNA species designated IFN alpha 1 and IFN alpha 2 were then used to screen a total human DNA gene library. At least 17 distinct genes have now been found which cross hybridise with the relevant probes and can be expressed. There may be several more pseudogenes which are not. Human IFN beta has also been cloned and possibly two different species of the gene isolated. IFN gamma DNA has also been isolated although only one chromosomal gene was found to correspond to it. Most studies have been with alpha IFN genes. These are transcribed into mRNA without any interruption of the reading sequence. No splicing step is required to produce mRNA ready for translation into protein. This indicates that there are no intervening sequences (introns) in the IFN and alpha DNA sequences. Both beta and gamma genes possess introns. The chromosomal location of these gene families has now been determined. The alpha family is closely linked and arranged in tandem on chromosome 9; the data on the chromosomal locations for beta and gamma genes are less clear cut. Currently, that for IFN gamma is thought to reside on chromosome 12.

Biochemical actions

The molecular mechanisms by which IFN exerts its effects on cells are extremely complex [4]. Cells exposed to IFN develop an anti-viral state in which the growth of RNA and DNA viruses is inhibited. This requires RNA and protein synthesis and is only temporary. Although a single mechanism may be responsible it is more likely that multiple sites of action are involved. These in turn cause many secondary biochemical changes within the cells. All biochemical activites are initiated by specific binding to surface receptors on the cell membrane. Alpha and beta IFN have the same receptor sites but the gamma receptor is separate. This may be important in view of the possible synergism between different IFN species. IFN is internalised and this is immediately followed by an increase in intracellular concentration of cyclic GMP. Some hours later cyclic AMP levels rise, the degree of elevation being related to the growth inhibitory effects. Reduced enzyme activity within IFN treated cells may be augmented or depressed, for example, increased prostaglandin synthesis has been observed.

Several new protein and mRNA types can be isolated from IFN treated cells and seem to be directly involved in the development of the anti-viral state. One pathway of action is related to protein kinase which may be switched on to increase the phosphorylation of intracellular molecules. This in turn may cause alterations in gene expression and DNA synthesis. The increase in intracellular 2-5A synthetase enzymes can be used as a marker for IFN stimulation. This results in inhibition of protein synthesis which is possibly the major contributor to the antiproliferative activities of IFN. In clinical practice, there is already some evidence that levels of 2-5A synthetase may be used to predict patient response to IFN therapy. In time this may be applied as part of a selection procedure to predict those patients with cancer who are likely to respond.

Two recent observations have suggested an interaction of IFN with products of oncogenes [5]. Oncogenes are segments of DNA coding for factors involved in cellular growth control. They are surprisingly well conserved during evolution suggesting a fundamental role in maintaining cell physiology. More recently, the function of the protein products of certain oncogenes has been elucidated; some act as growth factors or receptors for growth factors; others as protein kinases and a further group combine in a complex and non-covalent manner to nuclear structures. Differences in the expression of oncogenes have been found in normal and malignant cells, suggesting that they may have a pivotal role in the development of malignant disease.

In certain lymphoblastoid cell lines there is an abrupt reduction in c-*myc* transcript levels in IFN treated cells. The protein products of the c-*ras* and c-*src* genes in RT4 bladder carcinoma cells have also been found to be lowered with IFN treatment. These changes are accompanied by an inhibition of cell growth and replication. There is some controversy about the effects of interferon on c-*myc* expression. One group has demonstrated a decrease in the stability of the transcript presumably leading to reduced protein reduction. Others have shown a down regulation of gene expression. Recently sets of monoclonal antibodies to various oncogene proteins have been developed by peptide fragment immunisation. Immunoblotting techniques have been used to assess the level of oncogene product in tumour cell lines treated with interferon.

Immunological actions

It is known that IFN has a wide range of activity on the immune system. IFN is one of a series of communication molecules produced by the immune system allowing the constituent cells to gain information for stimulation and suppression [6] (Table 9.3). All the products listed in this table have similar molecular weights and indeed may have similar functions under certain circumstances. *In vivo* and *in vitro* studies have shown that IFN may both enhance and inhibit the immune response. For example, the injection of IFN before antigen inoculation in experimental model systems has been shown to increase the production of antibodies by B lymphocytes. The spectrum of antibody response may also be affected. The presence of IFN before antigen administration may reduce subsequent antibody production although its presence afterwards may enhance the same response.

Table 9.3 Immune control proteins

Protein	Origin cell	Action
IFN	ALL	ALL
IL1	MACRO	MACRO
IL2	T	TCGF
MIF	T	MACRO
MAF	T	MACRO
BCGF	MACRO	BCGF

MIF = migration inhibiting factor; MAF = macrophage activating factor; BCGF = B cell growth factor; and TCGF = T cell growth factor.

The effect of IFN on T lymphocytes is complex. Delayed hypersensitivity is markedly inhibited. Another class of lymphocyte, the natural killer (NK) cells, is also affected. Studies in mice and man show that interferon can agument NK cell function. This is thought to be mediated by an increase in the number of active NK cells. IFN may also mediate some of its general effects on the host by behaving as a lymphokine.

Clinical trials

Clinical effects of human IFNs have been investigated mainly using alpha IFN. Until 1978 the only preparation available was that from pooled buffy coat leucocytes produced in Helsinki by the Finnish Red Cross. In the mid 1970s Burroughs Wellcome in London invested considerable resources to obtain a lymphoblastoid line in tissue culture and to collect spent supernatants. There were many problems in the purification process until the advent of a monoclonal antibody that could be used on affinity columns. Human IFN beta has been manufactured for clinical trials both from human diploid fibroblasts and also from tumour cell lines. The first two IFNs produced by recombinant techniques were both alpha. There are problems of nomenclature resulting from the differences in the alpha gene family. Both alpha 2A and alpha 2B are available in large quantities of a highly purified form for clinical trials. Indeed, both are being used for the treatment of cancer in the UK.

Infectious diseases

Rational therapy for viral disease was clearly the main driving force in the early days of clinical IFN research. The first success in man was the demonstration of protection of volunteers from influenza and rhinovirus infection [7]. IFN was given as an intranasal spray and the symptoms of viral infection were reduced, provided treatment was given prior to viral infection. Whether prophylaxis against upper respiratory tract infections can become a reality by the use of exogenous IFN administration remains to be seen. There are several serious acute viral infections in which IFN has now been tried including rabies, hepatitis, herpes encephalitis and Lassa fever. The number of patients involved in these studies has been extremely small with no control groups. At present, no firm conclusions can be made as to the role of IFN in the management of these diseases. The major problem in patients with viral disease is that by the time signs and symptoms develop, the virus has already caused widespread intracellular damage. Therefore it seems over optimistic to expect systemic therapy at this stage to halt the pathology that has resulted. At best limitation of disease could occur.

In chronic viral infections the position is different [8]. There are several disease states such as chronic hepatitis, chronic cytomegalovirus, herpes simplex and Epstein–Barr virus infections where some patients develop a long term symbiosis with the virus. At certain phases in the viral life history clinical problems result as a result of the interaction of virus and host. A small percentage of patients who develop classical hepatitis for example go on to develop chronic active hepatitis. In this latter disease the virus persists in the liver causing continued degeneration of liver parenchyma with resulting cirrhosis. Virus particles persist in the blood and can be reduced or completely cleared by the administration of interferon. Many adults harbour cytomegalovirus. In patients that are immunosuppressed cytomegalovirus can be a major problem causing life-threatening illnesses. Again IFN has been shown to induce clinical and biological remissions in such patients (Table 9.4).

Table 9.4   The use of IFN in infectious diseases

Acute	Herpes simplex keratitis
	Herpes zoster in immunocompromised
Chronic	Cytomegalovirus
	Hepatitis B—chronic active hepatitis
	Viral papillomas
Prophylaxis	Vaccinia skin lesions
	Rhinovirus
	Coronavirus
	Influenza
Unproven	Adenovirus conjunctivitis
	Rabies
	HIV—pre AIDS
	Upper respiratory tract infection

Cancer

It is the anti-cancer potential of IFN that has led to the greatest recent interest in its clinical use. Relatively impure IFN was shown to have some effect in causing objective tumour regression in patients with myeloma, breast cancer and non-Hodgkin's lymphoma. However, the responses tended to be partial rather than complete, and transient in nature. The hope of pioneers in this field was that better tumour regression might be obtained if greater quantities of IFN were given to patients. The early preparations had serious side effects, principally fever, malaise and fatigue. Because of the impurity of the preparations used, the question remained as to whether these effects were intrinsic to IFN or a result of contaminants. There is no doubt that recombinant IFN has demonstrated objective regressions in certainly relatively rare tumour types. It is also clear that pure IFN has profound side effects (Table 9.5) which limit the dose. Careful pharmacokinetic studies have shown that doses beyond 20 million units per day over periods of greater than one month cannot be tolerated [9].

Table 9.5 The side effects of inteferon

Side/effect	Time of onset after start of treatment	Duration	Dose related
Pyrexia	1 hour	2–3 days	No
Myalgia	2–3 days	4–7 days	No
Nausea and vomiting	2–3 days	7–10 days	Yes
Headache	2–3 days	7–14 days	Yes
Lethargy	7–10 days	3–4 weeks	Yes
Anorexia and weight loss	10–14 days	3–4 weeks	Yes
CNS toxicity	21–28 days	7–14 days	Yes

Table 9.6 lists results from clinical trials using recombinant IFN in different cancer types. The most promising is hairy cell leukaemia, although whether survival is indeed prolonged is still in dispute. IFN may play some part in the management of other diseases, for example melanoma, renal cell carcinoma, chronic myeloid leukaemia, non-Hodgkin's lymphoma and Kaposi's sarcoma in patients with the acquired immunodeficiency syndrome [10].

TUMOUR NECROSIS FACTOR AND RELATED MOLECULES

The story of the tumour necrosis factor (TNF) goes back to 1891 when a New York physician William Coley, began giving patients mixtures

Table 9.6   Published tumour response rate (percentage) for alpha interferon

Type of cancer	CR	PR	LPR	NR
IFN possibly useful				
Hairy cell leukaemia	23	35	12	30
Myeloma	3	16	14	67
Non-Hodgkin's lymphoma	6	38	10	46
Kaposi's sarcoma	18	9	14	59
Renal cell carcinoma	31	43	5	21
Chronic meyloid leukaemia	30	25	9	36
IFN probably not useful				
Lung cancer	0	3	3	94
Breast cancer	0	3	7	90
Ovarian cancer	0	15	8	77
Colon cancer	0	11	16	73
Acute myeloblastic leukaemia	0	1	12	87

CR = clinical remission; PR = partial remission; LPR = less than partial response; and NR = no response.

of toxins from various bacteria. His rationale was that cancers sometimes regressed in patients after a severe bacterial infection such as erysipelas. The dramatic tumour responses he saw were later reported with evangelical zeal by his daughter and the whole subject of the anti-tumour effect of bacterial endotoxins heralded in the era of active immunotherapy [11]. *In vitro* experiments using the bacterial products themselves on a variety of tumour cell lines showed no evidence of cytotoxicity. This paradox was subsequently resolved by the discovery that endotoxins injected into suitably primed animals stimulated macrophages to produce a tumour necrosis factor and caused haemorrhagic necrosis in tumours. The serum of such animals was indeed cytotoxic to a range of cell lines. At the same time, several groups demonstrated that sensitised lymphocytes could also destroy tumour cells through soluble mediators—the lymphokines—including lymphotoxin (LT).

TNF and LT structure

Antibodies to partially purified TNF and LT provided evidence of structural differences between the two cancer toxins, both of which were able to distinguish between tumour and normal cell and destroy the former [12]. Although an intriguing new pair of selective tumour destroying agents had been discovered, experimentalists were plagued by their impurity. Batch to batch variation in biological assays and the lack of molecular characterisation precluded further analysis. Indeed, the observations were dismissed by some as an over-optimistic interpretation of confused data.

Against this background of doubt, the use of sophisticated biotechnology enabled the cloning of both TNF and LT. TNF was cloned from cDNA made from extracts of a human promyelocytic leukaemia line HL60 which produces large quantities of TNF upon appropriate stimulation. Amino acid sequence data from tryptic peptide analysis led to the construction of a 42 base oligodeoxynucleotide that was used to extract TNF cDNA from an HL60 library. From the structure of the cDNA, it was clear that TNF was made as a 157 amino acid precursor from which the amino terminal 76 segment was cleaved prior to secretion. The cleaved fragments may well represent an unusually long signal peptide and contain arginine and lysine dipeptide pairs of the kind often associated with the release of physiological peptides from precursor molecules. The TNF produced when the cDNA was expressed in E. coli was tested for biological activity and tumour necrosis was demonstrable with microgram quantities [13].

Lymphotoxin was purified from a phorbol ester-stimulated human lymphoblastoid cell line, its amino terminal 155 amino acids determined by microsequencing and the corresponding oligodeoxynucleotide synthesised [14]. This long probe was used to isolate a cDNA clone from which the complete LT sequence was derived. Again, a signal sequence was found, in this case 34 amino acids long. LT produced from the cDNA in E. coli has a clear antiproliferative effect on several human tumour cell lines but not on normal cells. Furthermore, in vivo experiments in mice showed destruction of several actively growing sarcomas.

Mechanism of action

Both TNF and LT can destroy tumour cells. The availability of structural data allowed an analysis of structure activity relationships. There is considerable similarity between the sequences of TNF and LT. Of the 157 amino acids of TNF, 44 are matched in LT. Many more amino acids show conservative changes. There are two well conserved regions within the molecules in addition to the hydrophobic C-terminals of both gene products. One conserved region perhaps binds to a cellular receptor, the others effecting cell destruction. There are many intriguing questions. What is the basis of selective tumour cell destruction? Do these toxins have to be released in the vicinity of a tumour or are they effective systemically? The availability of cloned genes allows the production of adequate quantities of these peptides for these questions to be addressed.

Clinical results

Only TNF has been evaluated in adequate clinical trial. The results have been extremely disappointing. Phase 1 studies have been carried out extensively using recombinant TNF of several types on both sides of the Atlantic and also in Japan. The first problem is the surprising toxicity of the agent. When a bolus of 10 mega units is given intravenously, rigors, fatigue, and anorexia occurs in most patients and in some toxic shock can develop. Stringent monitoring conditions are therefore essential during clinical investigation. In a recently published series of 18 patients with miscellaneous tumour types treated in a Phase 1 setting, only one well documented tumour response was seen. This patient who had non-Hodgkin's lymphoma showed partial regression of lymph node disease but only for a short period of time [15]. Similar data has been obtained in other series. In the 120 patients with documented disease that have been reported worldwide there is an overall response rate of less than 5%.

One surprising observation has been the rapidity with which TNF is cleared from the blood in patients. Pharmacokinetic data show a half-life of less than 30 minutes after intravenous bolus injection. For this reason, many studies have now moved to continuous infusion of TNF to determine whether achieving a higher serum concentration for a longer period of time may induce more tumour responses hopefully without increasing toxicity. Early data from these studies also seems disappointing.

Some intriguing observations have been made with a combination of TNF and other lymphokines, including the interferons. Only painstaking clinical research will reveal if these observations will alter in any way the management of patients with common tumours.

LYMPHOKINES

The cloning of genes coding for soluble products from lymphocytes which may be directly cytotoxic or may have specific regulatory roles on the immune response have also given rise to a new series of products for clinical trial. There are good indications that lymphokines can affect the complex network of the immune system, although the evidence for any anti-tumour effect is at present controversial.

Interleukin 1 (IL1) is a macrophage derived cytokine that activates certain T lymphocytes. In animal models it is shown to be a requirement for the production of cytotoxic T lymphocytes which have tumour destructive roles. Subsequently, it stimulates the production of interleukin 2 (IL2), a soluble protein involved in the maintenance of T cell growth and development. There are many other lymphokines that are currently being cloned that are involved in cell–cell communication within the immune system. There are also macrophage produced factors that directly inhibit cell growth. The physiological function of these soluble mediators is as yet unclear. Related to these lymphokines are thymus produced factors (Table 9.7). Again, the precise physiological role of these intriguing molecules remains unelucidated, although many experimental systems have shown a role for these factors in stimulating anti-tumour responses by the immune system.

LAK CELLS

One of the most enigmatic recent clinical observations has been of the tumour responses seen using lymphokine activated killer (LAK) cells. This work was pioneered by Steven Rosenberg at the National Cancer Institute (N.C.I.) in Washington. After a series of carefully controlled animal experiments, he went on to investigate the use of IL2 as a single agent in patients with several tumour types. In a series of 39 patients objective tumour regression was seen only rarely even with toxic doses of IL2. Other groups have claimed tumour responses, although most have been minor and of short duration.

In 1980 Rosenberg's group described the production of activated lymphoid cells which destroyed autologous tumour cells in both animal and human experiments. In a series of 27 patients with advanced metastatic cancer, no single tumour response was seen after the reinfusion of activated killer cells [16]. In 1984, 45 patients were treated at the N.C.I. with a combination of LAK cells and IL. A significant number of partial tumour responses were seen. This heralded in an era of extensive clinical investigation.

Table 9.7 Thymic hormones and their effects on T cell function and tumour growth

| Thymic factor | T cell effects | | Experimental tumour growth suppression |
	Help	Suppression	
Thymosin fraction 5	+	−	+
	+	−	−
Thymopoietin	−	+	+
Thymic hormonal factor (THF)	+	+	+
Thymostimulation	+	−	−
Facteur Thymique serique (FTS)	+	−	+

A major problem with LAK cell therapy is the complexity of the technology and the level of back up required. Furthermore, the toxicity determines that patients receive intensive care, with all its added costs, during and after the infusion of cells. There are now modifications to the LAK cell protocol which aim to reduce toxicity. Six large centres within the USA are evaluating the technique and similar investigations are in progress in many countries.

LAK cell administration

The largest series of patients treated in a consistent manner comes from the N.C.I. Patients were admitted to hospital and an intravenous infusion of 100 000 units of IL/kg body weight given every 8 hours. After a 2 day gap, patients underwent five daily leukaphereses with lymphocyte harvesting. LAK cells were prepared by separating lymphocytes on Ficoll-hypaque density gradients, harvesting and washing. Viable cells were incubated and treated with IL2 usually at a dose of 1000 units/ml for 3 days. After the fifth leukapheresis the patients received an infusion of the cells obtained from the first two extractions. The cells were administered intravenously through a central venous catheter over 30 minutes. In this way, cells that had been stimulated *in vitro* with IL2 for at least 4 days were given over a period of a week [16].

In the most recent update from the N.C.I. series, 106 patients received LAK cells with IL2. There were eight complete responses, 15 partial responses and ten minor responses [18]. The median duration of complete response was 10 months and 6 months amongst those patients with partial responses. Responses were seen in patients with renal cell carcinoma (53%), melanoma (27%), colorectal cancer (15%) and non-Hodgkin's lymphoma (100%—there were only two patients with this).

The mechanism of LAK/IL2 responses is unknown. Clearly the infused LAK cells may be destroying tumour cells directly or indirectly, recruiting other cells into this process by the release of soluble mediators. Most clinical research in this area is empirical, attempting to reproduce the tumour responses whilst reducing the toxicity. Until the precise molecular mechanisms are determined, it is difficult to see how logical progress in this area can occur.

CONCLUSIONS

One intriguing observation that comes from all clinical studies to date using various biological approaches has been the level of response and the disease spectrum in which responses are seen. There seems to be some special feature of renal cell cancer, melanoma, and non-Hodgkin's lymphoma that makes these neoplasms peculiarly sensitive to biological modifiers. It is interesting that these tumours often express strong tumour associated antigens and have been extensively studied by the use of monoclonal antibodies raised against cell surface molecules. The mode of action of most biological agents is still a mystery. However, the advent of purified preparations of so many molecules and our ability to combine them in novel ways has opened new avenues for clinical investigation. As we increase our understanding of growth control through the discovery of oncogenes and their products, it is likely that clinical benefit will be seen.

REFERENCES

1 Finter, M.V., (ed) *Interferons and Interferon Inducers*. Amsterdam: North Holland Publishing, 1973, 295–391.
2 Riordan, M.L. and Pitha-Rowe, P.M. Interferons and gene expression. In: Taylor-Papadimitriou, J. (ed) *Interferons and their Impact in Biology and Medicine*. Oxford: Oxford Medical Publications. 1985, 19–39.
3 Dijkman, S.R. and Billiau, A. An introduction to the genes of the interferon system. In: Taylor-Papadimitriou, J. (ed) *Interferons and their Impact in Biology and Medicine*. Oxford: Oxford Medical Publications. 1985.
4 Evinger, M., Rubinstein, M., Pestka, S. Antiproliferative and antiviral activities of human leucocyte interferons. *Arch Biochem Biophys*. 1981, **210**: 319–329.

5 Clemens, M. Interferons and oncogenes. *Nature.* 1985, **313**: 521–522.
6 Balkwill, F.R. The regulatory role of interferons in the human immune response. In: Taylor-Papadimitriou, J. (ed) *Interferons and their Impact in Biology and Medicine.* Oxford: Oxford Medical Publications, 1985, 61–62.
7 Merrigan, T.C., Read, S.E., Hall, T.S. *et al.* Inhibition of respiratory virus infection by locally applied interferon. *Lancet.* 1973, **1**: 563–567.
8 Merrigan, T.C., Rand, K.H. and Pollard, R.V. Human leucocyte interferon for the treatment of herpes zoster in patients with cancer. *New Engl J Med.* 1978, **298**: 981–987.
9 Smedley, H.M. and Wheeler, T.K. The toxicity of interferon. In: Sikora, K. (ed) *Interferon and Cancer.* New York: Plenum Press, 1983, 136–142.
10 Nethersell, A. and Sikora, K. Interferons and malignant disease. In: Taylor-Papadimitriou, J. (ed) *Interferons and their Impact in Biology in Medicine.* Oxford: Oxford Medical Publications, 1985, 127–145.
11 Sikora, K. Cancer toxins, genes cloned. *Nature.* 1984, **312**: 731–732.
12 Helson, L., Green, S., Carswell, E. and Old L.J. Effects of tumour necrosis factor on cultured human melanoma cells. *Nature.* 1975, **258**: 731–732.
13 Gray, P.W., Aggarwal, W. and Benton, B. *et al.* Cloning and expression of c-DNA for human lymphotoxin. *Nature,* 1984, **312**: 721–729.
14 Pennicka, D., Nedwin, G., Hayflink, E. *et al.* Human tumour necrosis factor: precursor structure, expression and homology to lymphotoxin. *Nature.* 1984, **312**: 724–729.
15 Selby, P. *Tumour Necrosis Factor in Man: Clinical and Biological Observations* (in press).
16 Rosenberg, S.A., Lotze M.T. and Mull, M. *et al.* Progress report on the treatment of 157 patients with advanced cancer using lymphokine activated killer cells and interleukin 2 or high dose interleukin 2 alone. *New England Journal of Medicine,* **316**: 889–897.

INDEX